Family Perspectives in Child and Youth Services

Family Perspectives in Child and Youth Services

David H. Olson
Editor

Routledge
Taylor & Francis Group
NEW YORK AND LONDON

Family Perspectives in Child and Youth Services has also been published as *Child & Youth Services*, Volume 11, Number 1 1988.

First published 1988 by The Haworth Press, Inc.

This edition published 2013 by Routledge
605 Third Avenue, New York, NY 10017
4 Park Square, Milton Park, Abingdon, Oxon OX14 4RN

Routledge is an imprint of the Taylor & Francis Group, an informa business

Library of Congress Cataloging-in-Publication Data

Family perspectives in child and youth services.

"Has also been published as Child & youth services, volume 11, number 1, 1988"—T.p. verso.
Includes bibliographical references and index.
1. Family social work. 2. Problem families—Counseling of. 3. Family psychotherapy. I. Olson, David H.
HV697.F365 1988 362.7'044 88-32006
ISBN 0-86656-850-6

ISBN 13: 978-0-86656-850-0 (hbk)

Family Perspectives in Child and Youth Services

CONTENTS

ABOUT THE EDITOR

David H. Olson, PhD, is Professor and former Director of the Graduate Program in Family Social Science at the University of Minnesota. He has extensive experience in the field of marital and family therapy and has published over ten books and 70 articles in this field. He developed the Circumplex Model of Marital and Family Systems and is committed to finding ways of integrating research, theory, and clinical practice. He is a Fellow in the American Association for Marriage and Family Therapy (AAMFT) and a Licensed Consulting Psychologist in the State of Minnesota. He is an associate editor or an editorial board member of eight professional family journals.

Foreword

This impressive collection of papers by David Olson and his colleagues provides additional form and substance to the effort, well under way, to extend the parameters of child and youth services to include families. Such a change is long overdue, and clinicians and administrators will find much of practical value here as they shift the orientation of their programs and services from child rescue to family support. Home visits, Parent training, and using child care workers as family workers are good ideas that are amply illustrated in the chapters to follow.

They constitute, however, but a portion of the many forms of family helping available to child and youth service practitioners. One hopes that these excellent papers will generate additional ideas and, hopefully, a few experiments on other formats for supporting and strengthening the diverse group of families that enter the child and youth services stream.

One hopes, finally, that more explicit ownership of the family work task in child and youth services will heighten the search for broader, more preventive interventions whose foci lie beyond the boundaries of individual families and extend to the wider community. It may just turn out that the most effective help and supports for at risk youth and families may come from the outside in, rather than the other way around.

James K. Whittaker
Seattle, Washington

Family Perspectives: An Overview

David H. Olson

Problems with children either begin or end up in the family. Because the family is both affected by and affects other family members, it is important that they be involved in the treatment of problem children. There is increasing clinical and empirical evidence that parents can be a useful, if not critical, resource in educational and therapeutic programs for helping problem children. Because many problem children have parents with problems, it might be more accurate to talk about problem parents than problem children. For this reason, it is even more important to help them become more effective parents.

I first became very aware of the powerful impact parents can have on their children when I was working at a residential treatment center for emotionally disturbed children. After several weeks of intensive treatment in the residential setting, we could see considerable progress in improving the child's social skills and adjustment. However, after a one day visit with his/her parents, many of the children regressed to their earlier level of functioning. This consistent pattern clearly demonstrated the power of the parents and stimulated interest among the staff as to how to make parents a more positive influence on the children.

Seeking useful ways of actively involving the family in the treatment of problem children is a central theme of this volume. This collection of papers focuses on two domains: "Family Assessment and Intervention Approaches" and "Parent Training and Prevention Approaches."

David H. Olson is affiliated with the Department of Family Social Science, University of Minnesota, 290 McNeal Hall, St. Paul, MN 55108.

FAMILY ASSESSMENT AND INTERVENTION APPROACHES

This section focuses on how family assessment and family intervention can be successfully utilized to treat problems with children and adolescents. First, a family model is presented which can be used for assessing family dynamics and for planning intervention. Secondly, a highly successful skill-building program is described which can improve parent-child relationships. Third, the value of home visits for motivating and involving family members is discussed and a study is summarized which supports their use. Lastly, the challenges and procedures of integrating family therapy into a traditional residential treatment center for children is clearly described.

In order to effectively help families, professionals need theoretical models that will help provide a framework for understanding and describing family dynamics. In the article, "Family Assessment and Intervention: The Circumplex Model of Family Systems," David Olson describes how systematic assessment and families can be accomplished. The Circumplex Model is described, which focuses on the three central dimensions of family cohesion, change (adaptability), and communication. Hypotheses have been derived from this model which have been systematically tested and validated. Clinical assessment can be done with either the self-report scale called FACES III or the Clinical Rating Scale, which an interviewer can use to summarize their evaluations. Education programs and therapeutic intervention can also be based on the Circumplex Model. In other words, the Circumplex Model provides a comprehensive understanding of a family system and enables practitioners to more adequately tailor their specific programs and interventions for families.

One of the most highly successful and effective skill building programs is called, Relationship Enhancement (RE) and it is described by their developers, Bernard Guerney and Louise Guerney. In their article entitled, "Building Relationship Skills in Families and Para-Family Teams," they contrast their educational skill-building model with the traditional medical model. Their program emphasizes communication and problem-solving skills, i.e., expressiveness, empathy, negotiation, conflict resolution and maintenance skills. Participants can both be family members where the child is either living or not living at home and para-family teams. Para-family teams include professionals who work together with the child and function as a pseudofamily. The children can be in foster care settings, residential treatment settings or in other placements outside the home. A variety of training formats can be adapted to the specific requirements demands of diverse settings. Built on systematic studies, this program has been demonstrated to be one of the most effective for building relationship skills in parent-child and other interpersonal relationships.

The multiple advantages of using home visits to increase the attendance and effectiveness of abusive and negligent parents in a parent training program is amply demonstrated in the article, "Home Visits: An Effective Strategy for Engaging the Involuntary Client" by Pallassana Balgopal, Michael Patchner, and Charles Henderson. In the early history of social work, home visits were an integral part of their professional activity. However, when visits became seen as intrusive and nonsupportive, the field shifted away from them as a resource for individuals and families with problems. The authors review a variety of goals which can be achieved by reintroducing home visits into all types of child and youth services.

They also conducted a systematic study of 34 abusing and neglecting parents and they found that home visits increased the participation level and information gained from the program. The training program involved eight weeks of two-hour parenting skills sessions held in a group setting. Home visits were introduced every two weeks. Based on their pre- and post-assessment, they found that the clients' attitudes towards home visits and attitudes towards the parent training sessions significantly improved. The authors, therefore, recommended that home visits increasingly be used as a way to improve the effectiveness of social services to individuals and families.

An excellent example of how general system theory can be applied both therapeutically in family therapy but also programmatically in terms of change within an organization is described in the paper by William Matthews and Janine Roberts. In the article, "The Entrance of Systems Family Therapy into a Residential Treatment Center" they review the successful step-by-step procedures which they used in introducing family system therapy into a traditional residential treatment center for adolescents.

They found that changing an organization like a residential treatment center has certain systematic similarities to trying to change a problem family. More specifically, both organizations and family systems resist change and have hierarchy and boundary issues which need to be understood and effectively dealt with. The paper describes how they systematically trained the staff and effectively integrated family therapy and system thinking into a residential treatment program.

PARENT TRAINING AND PREVENTION APPROACHES

The central themes of this section focus on utilizing parent training and emphasizing intervention with a goal toward prevention. Parents are typically underutilized in terms of programmatic intervention with a range of problems with children and adolescents. Because parents are potentially the most powerful resource in working with their children, they need to be increasingly and actively involved in any intervention program.

Family based services can not only help facilitate dealing with current child and adolescent problems, but training parents can also serve a critical preventive function. If parents are given useful communication and problem-solving skills, they can use these skills to deal with current parent-child issues. In addition, using these skills can also improve the quality of the parent-child relationship, thereby preventing future issues.

Family involvement can be integrated into all types of programs that work with and for children and adolescents. Marvin Bryce (1982) provides a useful model which illustrates the importance of family involvement in reducing cost and recidivism and how these dimensions vary across a range of services and programs (see Figure 1). In addition, Bryce (1982) has developed some useful principles regarding family involvement which are summarized in Table 1.

A comprehensive review of "Parent Training for Delinquency Prevention" by Mark Fraser, J. David Hawkins, and Matthew Howard describes the importance of parental training in increasing

FIGURE 1. A Model of Family-Based Programming

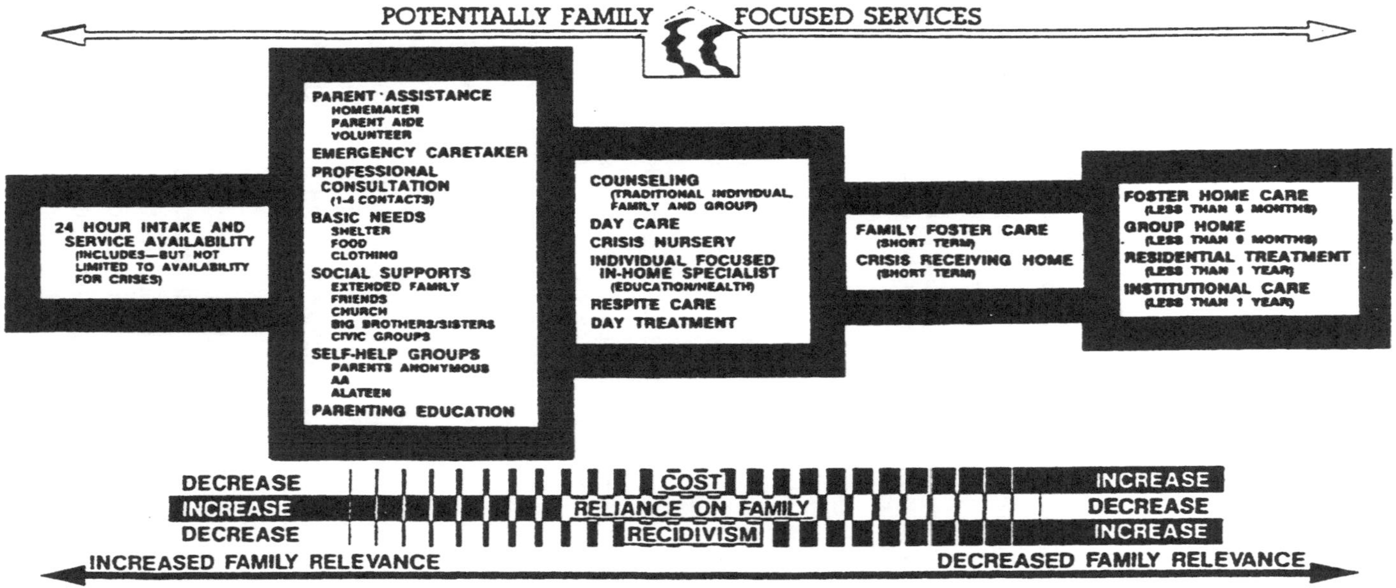

Reprinted from M. Bryce (1982) with permission.

TABLE 1. Principles of Placement Prevention and Family Reunification

1. A willingness to invest at least as much in a child's own family as society is willing to pay for out-of-home care for that child. This philosophy addresses the immense service vacuum which often exists between minimal services in the home and 24-hour care.

2. Service is as complete, comprehensive and intensive as necessary to reduce stress, increase constructive coping, assure safety, and to strengthen and maintain the family. Staff are available around the clock seven days a week.

3. The service setting is primarily the home, but includes problem solving efforts in the family's ecological system (where family interfaces with community).

4. Many of the programs provide help with any problem presented by the family or observed by the team. If the team does not have the expertise or resources needed, it arranges for or creates them.

5. Service agents are responsible for the family as the family is responsible for its members. There is maximum utilization of extended family, natural helping networks and other community resources.

6. The focus may be remedial and/or developmental. In programs with a developmental or primary prevention emphasis, rather than corrective, services are usually less intense.

7. Programs may be under social, health, or educational auspices.

8. The family is the service unit, the importance of cultural values to child development are recognized, and family priorities are respected.

9. Parents remain in charge of their family and participate in decision making, and family integrity is preserved.

Reprinted from M. Bryce (1982) with permission.

school achievement and decreasing disruptive and negative behaviors in adolescents. They describe family based educational programs for parents that emphasize the cognitive-behavioral orientation. These programs have consistently demonstrated to have short-term positive outcomes.

In their article, they provide a framework for evaluating parent training programs. They feel that there are four essential components that successful programs provide: (1) knowledge of parent-child relationships, (2) relationship and communication skills, (3) a system of rewards and mild punishment, (4) a verbal and written contract. Programs that build in these four components have tended to have the most success.

Problems in implementing parenting programs are also reviewed and ways of dealing with these issues are discussed. The issues include attrition, using peers as adjunctive therapists, the length of the program, whether to involve individuals and/or groups, cost of the training, the use of various types of communication and problem solving skills. Their review demonstrates that it is still unclear how much of this specific training generalizes to other aspects of the parent-child relationship or to other children and family members. It is also unclear how long these changes last and there is increasing need to attempt to make these programs more successful with high risk populations. However, it is clear that if family based programs are properly designed, they can reduce adolescent delinquent behaviors and improve parent-child relationships.

In the article, "Parents: Intervention Agents for Character Disorder and Juvenile Offenders," Magda Stouthamer-Loeber and Rolf Loeber first review relevant research articles on this topic. There is increasing empirical evidence regarding the impact of negative family dynamics on child and adolescent development. Their review focuses on the dimensions of family neglect, family conflict, deviant family value and family disruption.

Using an innovative evaluative approach entitled, "Relative Improvement Over Chance" (RIOC), they clearly demonstrate the significance of family dynamics over background on understanding and treating adolescent delinquent behaviors. They emphasize the value of family assessment in determining the specific issues and in developing an effective treatment plan. A variety of positive parental behaviors are described in terms of how they can help treat adolescent conduct disorders. Some of these interventions include parental supervision, improved communication skills, and increases in rewarding behaviors. They also provide some examples of how to use parents as change agents in the therapeutic process with adolescents for conduct disorders.

The paper, "Working with Families: Expanded Roles for Child Care Practitioners" by Karen Vander Ven provides a useful, three-level model of expertise in integrating the family into a variety of child care services. Level 1 involves direct work with children by younger people who are not yet parents. Services they can provide include information-giving, management by modeling, organized parent education and collaborator with parents. At Level 2, child care practitioners would include more experienced practitioners who would integrate a systems and ecological perspective into the parent-child relationship. They would also be more involved in developing parent programs that are relevant and focused on parenting skills. At Level 3, the practitioner would receive some clinical training which would enable them to provide more dynamically orientation education, skill building programs for families and knowledge about family therapy. The article closes with a summary of recommendations for enhancing the role of child care practitioners so that they can work more effectively with parents.

In the final paper entitled, "Family Based Services: Preventive Intervention" by Marvin Bryce, the value of home based programs is emphasized. The child welfare policy of placing children outside the home is reviewed historically, politically and programmatically. Since the 1980s there has been an increasing interest in family based programs which has been stimulated by congressional mandates and increasing financial incentives for these types of programs. The family based preventive approach was initiated more in the private sector but is increasingly moving into publicly funded programs. He reviews numerous programs which have been successful in reducing the out-of-home placement and decreasing child institutionalization. He also describes problems which have limited the public agencies adopting family programs and illustrates how these problems can be effectively overcome. He emphasizes that family based programs will increase as financial incentives are built into legislative and agency programming.

REFERENCE

Bryce, M. (1982). Family based services: Relevance for prevention. *Prevention Report*. Oakdale, IA: National Resource Center on Family Based Services, University of Iowa.

FAMILY ASSESSMENT AND INTERVENTION APPROACHES

Family Assessment and Intervention: The Circumplex Model of Family Systems

David H. Olson

ABSTRACT. This paper describes how the Circumplex Model can be used for systematic assessment of a marital and family system. The three dimensions in the Circumplex are cohesion, change (adaptability) and communication. A variety of hypotheses have been derived and tested which validate the Circumplex Model. Clinical assessment and research can utilize the self-report scale, FACES III or the Clinical Rating Scale can be used to evaluate the family based on a clinical interview. A clinical evaluation of a problem family using FACES III and Clinical Rating Scale demonstrates the value of the tools for family assessment and treatment planning. The paper reflects the continuing attempt to further develop the Circumplex Model and more adequately bridge research, theory and practice.

The Circumplex Model of Marital and Family Systems was developed in an attempt to bridge the gap that typically exists between research, theory and practice. One major approach used to bridge

---

David H. Olson is affiliated with the Department of Family Social Science, University of Minnesota, 290 McNeal Hall, St. Paul, MN 55108.

This article has also appeared in a revised version in *Journal of Psychotherapy & the Family* 4(1/2) 1988.

this gap has been the systematic development of both a self-report and clinical rating scale based on the Circumplex Model. Both the self-report scale, called FACES III, and the Clinical Rating Scale have been revised several times to increase their reliability, validity and clinical utility.

A variety of hypotheses have been developed and tested using the Circumplex Model. Some of the research has focused on the relationship between family symptoms and types of family systems. Recent studies are investigating changes in family types before and after treatment and change during the treatment process.

In addition to its value in research projects, the Circumplex Model can also be used in clinical practice. Clinically, it can be used for assessing marital and family systems and for planning treatment intervention. In addition to identifying types of family systems, work is currently being done to describe the type of therapeutic techniques and interventions that are most and least effective with various types of systems.

FAMILY COHESION, ADAPTABILITY (CHANGE), AND COMMUNICATION

Family cohesion, adaptability, and communication are three dimensions of family behavior that emerge from a conceptual clustering of over 50 concepts developed to describe marital and family dynamics. Although some of these concepts have been used for decades (power and roles, for instance), many of the concepts have been developed recently by individuals observing problem families from a general systems perspective (pseudomutuality, double binds).

After reviewing the conceptual definitions of many of these concepts, it became apparent that despite the creative terminology, the terms were conceptually similar and dealt with highly related family processes. One family process had to do with the degree to which an individual was separated from or connected to his or her family system and was called family cohesion. The second dimension was family adaptability, which focused on the extent to which the family system was flexible and able to change. The third dimension focused on family communication between various members.

Family cohesion is defined as the emotional bonding that family members have toward one another. Within the Circumplex Model, some of the specific concepts or variables that can be used to diagnose and measure the family cohesion dimensions are: emotional bonding, boundaries, coalitions, time, space, friends, decision making, and interests and recreation.

There are four levels of cohesion, ranging from disengaged (very low) to separated (low to moderate) to connected (moderate to high) to enmeshed (very high) (see Figure 1). It is hypothesized that the central levels of cohesion (separated and connected) make for optimal family functioning. The extremes (disengaged or enmeshed) are generally seen as problematic.

Many couples and families that come for treatment often fall into one of these extremes. When cohesion levels are high (enmeshed systems), there is too much consensus within the family and too little independence. At the other extreme (disengaged systems), family members "do their own thing," with limited attachment or commitment to their family. In the model's central area (separated and connected), individuals are able to experience and balance between these two extremes and are able to both be independent from and connected to their families.

Family adaptability is defined as the ability of a marital or family system to change its power structure, role relationships, and relationship rules in response to situational and developmental stress. In order to describe, measure, and diagnose couples on this dimension, a variety of concepts have been taken from several social science disciplines, with heavy reliance on family sociology. These concepts include: family power (assertiveness, control, discipline), negotiation styles, role relationships and relationship rules.

The four levels of adaptability range from rigid (very low) to structured (low to moderate) to flexible (moderate to high) to chaotic (very high) (see Figure 1). As with cohesion, it is hypothesized that central levels of adaptability (structured and flexible) are more conducive to marital and family functioning, with the extremes (rigid and chaotic) being the most problematic for families as they move through the family life cycle.

Basically, adaptability focuses on the ability of the marital and family system to change. Much of the early application of systems

FIGURE 1. CIRCUMPLEX MODEL: SIXTEEN TYPES OF MARITAL AND FAMILY SYSTEMS

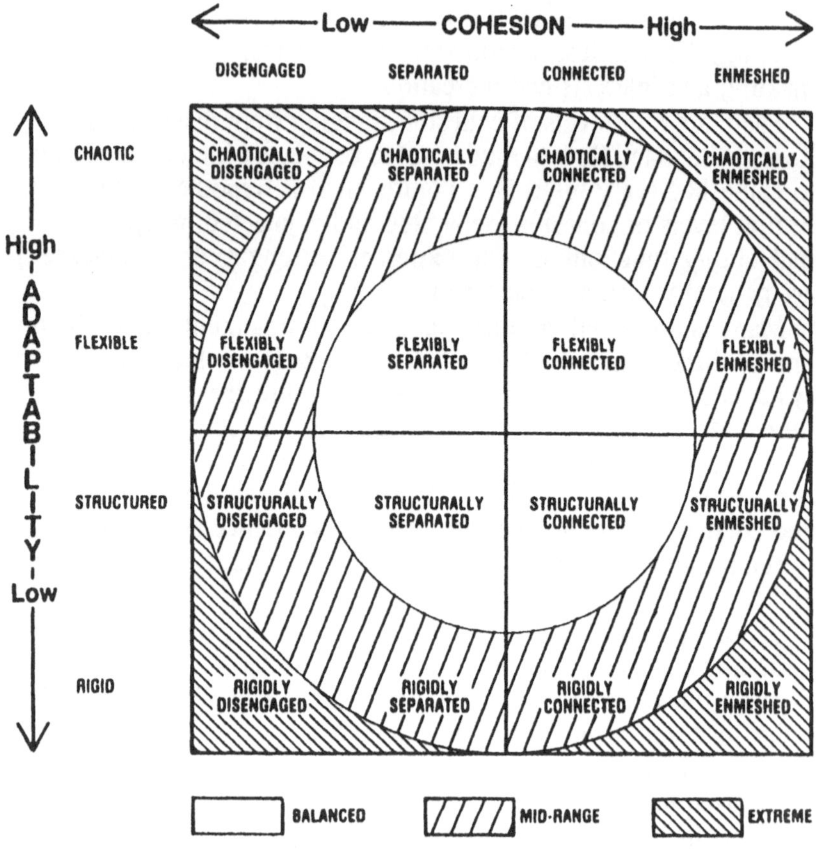

theory to families emphasized the rigidity of the family and its tendency to maintain the status quo. Until the work of theorists, the importance of potential for change was minimized. Couples and families need both stability and change and the ability to change when appropriate distinguishes functional couples and families from others.

Family communication is the third dimension in the Circumplex

Model, and is considered a facilitating dimension. Communication is considered critical for facilitating couples and families to move on the other two dimensions. Because it is a facilitating dimension, communication is not graphically included in the model along with cohesion and adaptability.

Positive communication skills (i.e., empathy, reflective listening, supportive comments) enable couples and families to share with each other their changing needs and preferences as they relate to cohesion and adaptability. Negative communication skills (i.e., double messages, double binds, criticism) minimize the ability of a couple or family members to share their feelings and, thereby, restrict their movement on these dimensions.

Theoretical Models of Family Systems

A variety of other theoretical models that have focused independently on variables related to the cohesion, adaptability, and communication dimensions. Most of these models have been developed in the last 10 years by individuals having a system perspective of family. Evidence regarding the value and importance of these three dimensions is the fact that these therapists quite independently concluded that the variables they selected were critical for understanding and treating marital and family systems.

Table 1 summarizes the work of 10 theorists who have worked on describing marital and family systems. Most of the recent theorizing about family dynamics and intervention has been strongly influenced by general systems theory. Current work has focused on describing both clinical and nonclinical families or has been concerned with clinical intervention.

Marital and Family Adaptability (Change)

Adaptability measures the amount of change in a marriage or family. Marriages and families can range from having a rigid and authoritarian leader to being chaotic with erratic or limited leadership. A rigid relationship is where one person is highly controlling. The roles are strictly defined and the rules do not change. A structured relationship is overall less rigid. Leadership is somewhat less

Table 1: Theoretical Models Using Cohesion, Adaptability, and Communication

	Cohesion	Adaptability	Communication
Beavers & Voeller (1983)	Centripetal Centrifugal	Adaptability	
Benjamin (1977)	Affiliation	Interdependence	
Epstein, Bishop & Levin (1978)	Affective Involvement	Behavior Control Problem-Solving Roles	Communication Affective Responsiveness
French & Guldera (1974)		Capacity to change Power	
Gottman (1979)	Validation	Contrasting	
Kantor & Lehr (1975)	Affect Dimension	Power Dimension	
L'Abate (1985)	Intimacy	Power	
Leary (1957) & Constantine (1986)	Affection Hostility	Dominance Submission	
Leff & Vaughn (1985)	Distance	Problem Solving	
Parsons & Bales (1955)	Expressive Role	Instrumental Role	
Reiss (1981)	Coordination	Closure	

authoritarian and controlling, which is shared between the parents. Roles are stable, but there is some sharing of roles. There are few rule changes, but not a lot of change. A flexible relationship is even less rigid. Leadership is more equally shared. Roles are sometimes shared and rules could change. A chaotic relationship has erratic or limited leadership. Decisions are impulsive and not well thought-out. Roles are unclear and often shifted from person to person.

Based on the Couple & Family Map, very high levels of change (Chaotic) and very low levels of change (Rigid) might be problematic for a marriage and family. On the other hand, relationships having moderate scores (Structured and Flexible) are able to balance some change and some stability in a more functional way. Although there is no absolute best level for any relationship, many relationships may have problems if they always function at either extreme of the Map (Rigid and Chaotic) (see Figure 2).

Marital and Family Cohesion (Togetherness)

Cohesion measures the amount of togetherness in a marriage or family. Marriages and families range from being very close or enmeshed, to being very distant or disengaged from each other.

A disengaged relationship often has extreme emotional separateness. There is little involvement between the couple or a family member and a lot of personal separateness and independence. People often do their own thing and have separate interests.

A separated relationship has some emotional separateness but it is not as extreme as the disengaged system. While time apart is important, there is some time together and some joint decisions. Activities and interests are generally separate but a few are shared. A connected relationship has some emotional closeness and loyalty in the relationship. Time together is more important than time apart to be by oneself. There is an emphasis on togetherness. While there are separate friends, there are also friends shared by the couple. There are often shared interests.

In the enmeshed relationship, there is an extreme amount of emotional closeness and loyalty is demanded. Persons are very dependent on each other and reactive to one another. There is a general lack of personal separateness and little private space is permitted. The energy of the persons is mainly focused inside the marriage or family and there are few outside individual friends or interests.

Based on the Circumplex Model, high levels of cohesion (Enmeshed) and low levels of cohesion (Disengaged) might be problematic for relationships. On the other hand, relationships having moderate scores (Separated and Connected) are able to balance being alone together in a more functional way. Although there is no absolute best level for any relationship, some may have problems if they always function at either extreme of the Map (Disengaged and Enmeshed).

Figure 2: CIRCUMPLEX MODEL - Couple & Family Map

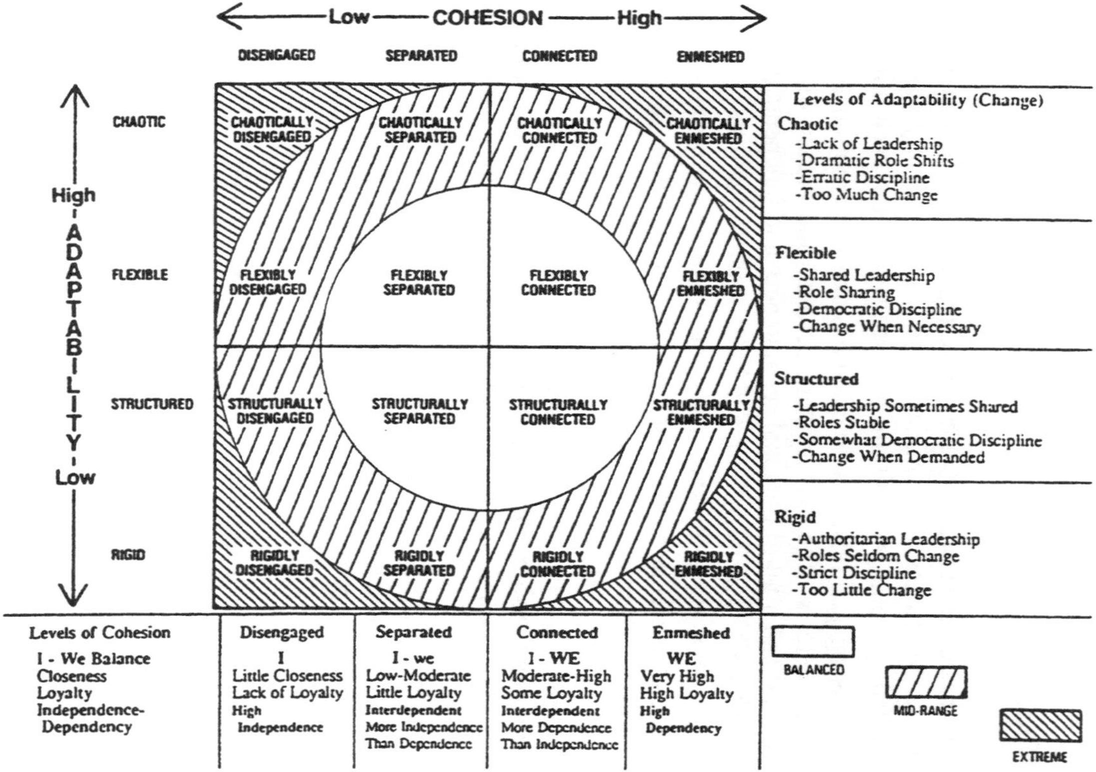

CIRCUMPLEX MODEL: COUPLE AND FAMILY MAP

Another way to consider the Circumplex Model is as a map of 16 types of couple and family relationships, in other words a Couple Map and a Family Map. The Couple Map is used to describe 16 Types of Marriage. The Family Map is used to describe a person's Family of Origin.

The Family Map is important because people often tend to recreate their past family system in their marriage. People either recreate the type of family system they had as a child or they react by doing the opposite. Thus, if a couple came from two quite different family systems, on either cohesion or adaptability, this may create some conflict for them as a couple.

Type of Marriage, as illustrated on the Couple Map, is important for the development of a couple. Couples need to balance their levels of separateness-togetherness on cohesion and their levels of stability-change on adaptability. These levels can be adjusted by a couple to achieve a level that is acceptable to each person.

There are several ways couples can have difficulty in balancing these levels of cohesion and adaptability. First, one or both partners might not like the levels of cohesion or adaptability they currently have in their relationship. That is, one person might feel the relationship is too low on cohesion (separated type) and the other might feel their partner is too smothering (enmeshed type).

Secondly, couples might disagree on how they actually see their marriage. One might see their marriage on cohesion as disengaged and the other might see it as connected. In terms of adaptability, one person might see their marriage as rigid and the other might see it as flexible. If a couple disagrees too much, it will often reflect dissatisfaction with their current relationship.

Couples can make deliberate attempts to change their marriage on cohesion and adaptability. This is important to do to keep the marriage more satisfying. Couples need to discuss how they each see the relationship and to explore possible directions for change. This will enable couples to have some goals to make their marriage more mutually satisfying.

Balanced versus Extreme Types

An important distinction in the Circumplex Model is between balanced and extreme types of couple and family relationships. There are four balanced types that are separated or connected levels on cohesion and structured or connected on adaptability. The four extreme types are disengaged or enmeshed on cohesion and rigid or chaotic on adaptability. Figure 3 describes in some detail the characteristics of the four balanced relationships and a description of the four extreme relationships: chaotically disengaged, chaotically enmeshed, rigidly disengaged and rigidly enmeshed.

Circumplex Types as Illustrated by the Movies

Movies often provide excellent examples of Extreme types of couple and family relationships because these are more dynamically and dramatically interesting. Table 2 lists movies that illustrate the four Extreme types and the Cosby TV Show illustrates how balanced families operate. A brief description of each movie and Extreme type is given below.

"The Great Santini": Rigidly Enmeshed

This is a military family, both inside and out. Dad (played by Robert Duvall) is a colonel in the Marines and wants to run his family the same way. He is rigidly enmeshed especially with his oldest son, whom he wants to follow in his footsteps into the Marines. On top of that, the son is supposed to excel in sports. For him the son's achievement means his achievement.

But the father cannot just cheer his son from the sidelines. In a one-on-one home basketball game, the son beats the father and the father cannot take the defeat, saying he must win by at least two points. He bullies the son, trying to get him to cry. He bounces the ball off the kid's forehead in a mocking, confrontive manner, trying to get his son to admit of weakness after his son has just beaten him.

None of the other kids have ever beaten the father at any sport, not at ping-pong, checkers, cards, anything. Dad always has to win. So when the sons beats him, Dad can't take it. He ridicules his son, trying to get him to cry so he will feel superior again.

Figure 3: CIRCUMPLEX MODEL - Balanced and Extreme Types

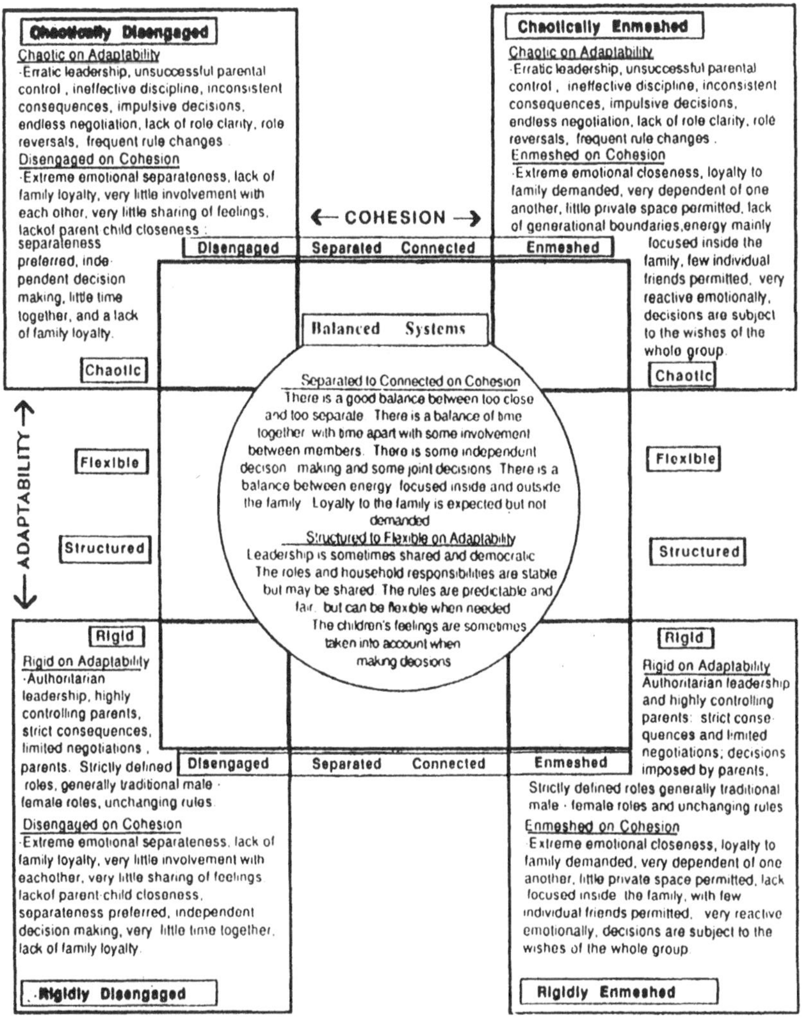

The mother acts in a typical codependent way. She makes excuses for him, defends him to the kids, and is careful not to cross him.

Dad primarily ignores his two daughters and his youngest son. The second oldest child, a daughter, tries to sarcastically engage him, wondering if she can be a full "Meecham" (the family name),

Table 2: Circumplex Types As Illustrated By Movies

Circumplex Types	Movies/TV
Rigidly Enmeshed	Great Santini
Rigidly Disengaged	Ordinary People
Chaotically Disengaged	Shoot the Moon
Chaotically Enmeshed	Who's Afraid of Virginia Woolf?
Balanced Type	Cosby TV Show

since she doesn't have a jump shot . . . or if she is destined to only be a "simple, single-celled Meecham," like in biology.

This family has a very rigid system. Rules are set down and strictly enforced by Dad. There will be no deviance from them, no whimpering or complaining.

This is also a very enmeshed system. Loyalty is demanded. The son's achievements are a reflection on Dad . . . and an extension of Dad's ego. There is no letting go of Dad. He is the center of the family. He sets the tone. If he is up, the family is up, if he is down, the family better watch out. This is an enmeshment based on intimidation, not on affection or even feigned affection. But the intimidation works. Mom, who of course has lived with Dad the longest, has the typical way of putting herself last to keep Dad happy, and does not question it.

"Ordinary People": Rigidly Disengaged

The other extreme of the cohesion dimension is the disengaged family from the movie, "Ordinary People." There is rigidity in this pleasant suburban family with mother (played by Mary Tyler Moore) and husband (played by Donald Sutherland). Unlike the angry, authoritarian rigidity of the Meechams in "The Great Santini," this is a kind of passive, controlling, but outwardly pleasant rigidity. It's a rigidity that must maintain a good appearance to all outsiders.

This rigidity was born in part out of a need to survive the loss of the oldest son in a boating accident on Lake Michigan, just a few months before the beginning of the story. Their son, Buck, was the star of the family: handsome, charming, excellent student, star athlete, and now tragically gone. His death has left an emptiness in mother that is defended against through her rigidity and disengagement, which moves the rest of the family in this direction as well.

There is a good deal of emotional controlling, strictly defined roles and unchanging rules . . . especially the rules about what feelings can be openly discussed. The surviving son, who has attempted suicide over his guilt surrounding the boating accident, cannot talk about his feelings in the family because of the implicit rules forbidding such intimate and painful self-disclosure.

Likewise, the disengagement in this family is painfully apparent. Feelings are not discussed and a distance is carefully maintained to prevent any future grief. There are attempts by the son and the husband to make contact with mother, but they fail.

Near the end of the movie, the mother wakes up in the middle of the night and finds her husband not at her side. She does downstairs and finds him sitting in the dining room, in the dark, crying softly to himself. He says he doesn't think he knows her anymore. She is so cautious. When Buck died, a part of her died. He does not know the woman who is left behind. And he is not sure he loves her anymore. Without another word, she goes upstairs and begins packing her suitcase to leave. There is a brief moment when she gasps, and nearly cries. She regains control, resumes packing and leaves.

Both of these families are rigid and the rigidity affects the degree of emotional closeness in these families. In "The Great Santini," the rigidity serves the purpose of controlling the level of enmeshment. The demands for family loyalty, the lack of individuation, and emotional reactivity are thrust upon the system by the power they give to the father who dictates the rules of the family: what people should do, how they should perform, and what their level of importance should be within his rigid view of the family.

In "Ordinary People," the rigidity serves the purpose of maintaining emotional disengagement in order to prevent the surfacing of the grief and guilt over the loss of the oldest son. It's as if Mom is keeping everyone at arm's length by emotionally stiff-arming her son and husband. And it's Mom's rigidity that both husband and son respond to by finally giving up in despair for any real attempt at emotional contact.

"Shoot the Moon": Chaotically Disengaged

This is a family falling apart. Dad (played by Albert Finney) has been having an affair. He's been trying to keep it from the family, but his oldest daughter is suspicious and listens in on a conversation he has with his lover from an extension at home. He has never called his lover from a phone at home before. But he is desperately in love and beginning to get careless.

His wife (played by Diane Keaton) has been suspicious for some time, but has not confronted him on it. However, his excuses for "working late" wear pretty thin and she finally does confront him and a dish-breaking fight ensues. He suggests he should leave and she says she packed his bag last night.

The disengagement of the couple really shows in these early scenes of the movie. They have not been connected in a long time as their estrangement has become more extensive. When he finally does move out, the chaos in the family system takes its turn.

The oldest daughter, Julie, takes over Mom's role. Mom sleeps late, buries her head under the pillow, moans, and turns over to try to escape her pain. This happens to a woman who before was never tired and was always patient and had time for her four daughters. In a scene typical of the family chaos, the oldest daughter is trying to make breakfast, talk on the phone to a doctor's office to make an appointment for one of her sisters who sprained her foot, and at the same time yelling upstairs at her sisters to get downstairs for breakfast, and burning the toast. The sisters yell back down that they don't want her breakfast (that she so carefully has tried to prepare) . . . and so she yells back at them that she doesn't need this . . . , throws the frying pan of scrambled eggs into the kitchen sink and heads out to the school bus.

Dad is waiting at the end of the driveway to pick them up in his car to take them to school himself . . . trying to overcome his guilt and spend some time with his daughters at the same time. The oldest, parentified daughter just walks around his car and gets onto the bus without saying a word to him. The bus pulls out and she can be seen looking through the bus window . . . crying.

This couple has been disengaged for some time. And the dad is also disengaged from his daughters. The mom has been close to her daughters before the separation . . . but even she gets disengaged from them – through her depression. The rules and roles are all up for grabs in this family. The father has left, the mother is depressed and unable to function, and the oldest daughter has taken over some of the parenting roles . . . while still wanting to have a mother and father care for her and be in charge.

"Who's Afraid of Virginia Woolf?": Chaotically Enmeshed

This is a good example of a classically chaotically enmeshed alcoholic system. George (Richard Burton) and Martha (Elizabeth Taylor) have a dependent, love-hate relationship bound together by unseen but powerful forces of mutual dependence and kept tolerable for each through the numbing and disorienting properties of alcohol.

George is an associate professor of English at a small college and Martha is the president's daughter. Martha and her father were impressed with George at first, but have become increasingly disenchanted with him over time. Martha thinks he's a "nothing," a wash-up and an enormous disappointment. And George things Martha is a monster, whom he said used to howl and claw at the turf outside his window when he first came to the college. So he married her, he said, in order to get some work done.

They cannot let go of each other. They fight dirty: they know where to attack each other's vulnerability and don't hesitate to do so. To George, Martha is a promiscuous, liquor-ridden monster who never hesitates to make a fool of herself. And to Martha, George is a weak-willed, pretentious, academic flop. They even share a secret, a mutual fantasy of a son. Since they were never able to have children, they created one. They even created a history for him and obviously invested a good deal of their hopes and dreams in this fantasy.

But one night, in an extended drunken battle when two guests come over after a faculty party, the secret gets disclosed. And for a while it looks like their enmeshed relationship will come unraveled through the chaotic fighting during the course of an endless nightmare of fighting. They break mutually-agreed-upon rules, but manage to stick together in the end, even though it looks as though they will destroy each other.

Their extreme enmeshment and dependency keeps them together when it looks like their system chaos will tear them apart. But they survive the pain of their enmeshment dependency by using alcohol or fantasy when the pain gets too intolerable.

HYPOTHESES DERIVED FROM THE CIRCUMPLEX MODEL

One of the assets of a theoretical model is that hypotheses can be deduced and tested in order to evaluate and further develop the model. The following are hypotheses derived from the model.

I. Couples/families with balanced (two central levels) cohesion and adaptability will generally function more adequately across the family life cycle than those at the extreme of these dimensions.

An important issue in the Circumplex Model relates to the concept of balance. Even though a balanced family system is placed at the two central levels of the model, it should not be assumed that these families always operate in a "moderate" manner. Being balanced means that a family system can experience the extremes on the dimension when appropriate but that they are not typically function at these extremes for long periods of time.

Families in the balanced area of the cohesion dimension allow family members to experience being both independent from and connected to their family. Both extremes are tolerated and expected, but the family does not continually function at the extreme. Conversely, extreme family types tend to function only at the extreme and are not encouraged to change the way they function as a family. This leads to Hypothesis II.

II. Balanced family types have a larger behavioral repertoire and are more able to change compared with extreme family types.

Integrating Normative Expectations of Families

Although a curvilinear relationship is generally predicted, some important qualifications must be made in terms of the normative expectations and cultural bias of Hypothesis I. Hypothesis III states:

III. If the normative expectations of a couple or family support behaviors extreme on one or both of the Circumplex dimensions, they will function well as long as all family members accept these expectations.

The normative expectations in our culture provide two conflicting themes that can create problems for couples and families. One theme is that family members are expected to do things together as a family. Yet, the second theme encourages individuals to "do their own thing" and develop themselves. The theme of independence becomes more prominent as children approach adolescence and has taken on greater importance for increasing numbers of women in our culture. As a result, many American families find that a balance of the two themes has become a difficult issue.

Families in our culture still vary greatly in the extent to which they encourage family closeness and individual development. Although most parents would prefer their children to develop values and ideas similar to theirs, most parents also want their children to become somewhat autonomous and differentiated from the family system.

A sizable minority of families, however, have normative expectations that strongly emphasize family togetherness. Their family norms emphasize emotional and physical togetherness, and they strive for high levels of consensus and loyalty. Some ethnic groups in this country such as Slovak-American, Puerto Rican, and Italian families, and religious groups such as the Amish and Mormans have high expectations regarding family togetherness.

These expectations are also common, but less predominant, in many other American families regardless of ethnic or religious orientation. Many of these families could be described as extreme on the cohesion dimension (i.e., enmeshed), and they function well as long as all family members are willing to go along with those expectations.

Family Communication as a Facilitating Dimension

Communication is a critical dimension related to the Circumplex Model because it facilitates movement on the two dimensions. This leads to two specific hypotheses linking communication to balanced types and change on cohesion and adaptability.

V. Balanced couples/families will tend to have more positive communication skills than extreme families.

VI. Positive communication skills will enable balanced couples/families to change their levels of cohesion and adaptability more easily than those at the extremes.

In general, positive communication skills are seen as helping marital and family systems facilitate and maintain a balance on the two dimensions. Conversely, negative communication skills impede from moving into the central areas and thereby, increase the probability that extreme systems will remain extreme.

Positive communication skills include the following: sending clear and congruent messages, empathy, supportive statements, and effective problem-solving skills. Conversely, negative communication skills include the following: sending incongruent and disqualifying messages, lack of empathy, nonsupportive (negative) statements, poor problem-solving skills, and paradoxical and double-binding messages. Although many studies have investigated communication and problem-solving skills in couples and families, these studies have not specifically tested the relationships of these skills to the hypotheses derived from the Circumplex Model.

Family Development and the Circumplex Model

VII. To deal with situational stress and developmental changes across the family life cycle, balanced families will change their cohesion and adaptability, whereas extreme families will resist change over time.

This hypothesis deals with change in the family system to deal with stress or to accommodate changes in family members, particularly as family members alter their expectations. The Circumplex

Model is dynamic in that it assumes that couples and families will change types, and it hypothesizes that change can be beneficial to the maintenance and improvement of family functioning.

When one family member desires change, the family system must somehow deal with that request. For example, increasing numbers of married women want to develop more autonomy from their husbands (cohesion dimension) and also want more power and equality in their relationships (adaptability dimension). If their husbands are unwilling to understand and change in accordance with these expectations, the marriages will probably experience increasing levels of stress.

Another common example of changing expectations occurs when a child reaches adolescence. Like the wife in the previous example, adolescents often want more freedom, independence, and power in the family system.

The Circumplex Model allows one to integrate systems theory with family development, a proposal made more than a decade ago by Reuben Hill. Building on the family development approach, as described by Hill and Rodgers, it is hypothesized that families must change as they deal with normal transitions in the family. It is expected, therefore, that the stage of the family life cycle and composition of the family will have considerable impact on the type of family system.

It is first of all hypothesized that at any stage of the family life cycle, there will be a diversity in the types of family system as described in the Circumplex Model. In spite of this diversity, it is predicted that at different stages of the family life cycle many of the families will cluster together in some types more frequently than in others. For example, it would be predicted that premarital couples would tend toward the high range on cohesion (enmeshed and connected) and toward the lower range on adaptability (structured and rigid). In other words, they would fall into the lower right quadrant of the Circumplex Model.

The model is dynamic in that it assumes that changes can occur in family types over time. Families are free to move in any direction that the situation, stage of the family life cycle, or socialization of family members may require. A look at a couple illustrates the dynamic nature of the model.

Steve and Sally were married and developed a flexibly enmeshed marriage. Three years after their marriage, they became parents, and Sally resigned from her teaching job. Because of the dependency needs of their son and their own desire for mutual support in this transition period, their family became structurally connected.

However, when Sally's and Steve's son became a teenager, their family moved from being connected to being more separated on cohesion. Sally started pursuing a career, and both parents experienced a good deal of "consciousness-raising" about sex roles through the media and through involvement in several growth groups. Because of their son's needs for more autonomy at this age, as well as the parents' separate career interests, they began operating at a lower level of cohesiveness.

Furthermore, the family power structure shifted from being husband-dominant to a more shared pattern. They moved on adaptability from a structured type to a flexible type. Sally exercised much more control in the relationship than previously, and the couple were struggling, almost on a weekly basis, to redefine the rules and role definitions that will govern their relationship. Although they occasionally yearn for the security of their earlier, more structured relationship, both found the challenge in this more flexible relationship style.

In short, their family could be described as flexibly separated of the family life cycle. This brief case history illustrates the dynamic nature of the model, which allows for movement within reasonable limits. It also seeks to recognize diverse values and legitimize the diverse organizational ideals of families. None of the four balanced types in the inner circle is designated as "the ideal" at any given stage of the family life cycle, but all are more functional than the extreme types, especially with families at the adolescent stage.

STUDIES VALIDATING THE CIRCUMPLEX MODEL

Balanced versus Extreme Families

A central hypothesis derived from the model is that balanced couples/families will function more adequately than extreme couples/families. This hypothesis is built on the assumption that families extreme on both dimensions will tend to have more difficulties functioning across the life cycle. This assumes a curvilinear relationship on the dimensions of cohesion and adaptability. This means that too little or too much cohesion or adaptability is seen as dysfunctional to the family system. However, families that are able to balance between these two extremes seem to function more adequately.

To test the major hypothesis that balanced family types are more functional than extreme types, a variety of studies have been done focusing on range of emotional problems and symptoms in couples and families. A recent study by Clark (1984) focused on families with schizophrenics, neurotics, families who had therapy sometime in their past, and a no-therapy control group (see Figure 4). In general, he found a very high level of extreme families in the neurotic

FIGURE 4: Problem Families:

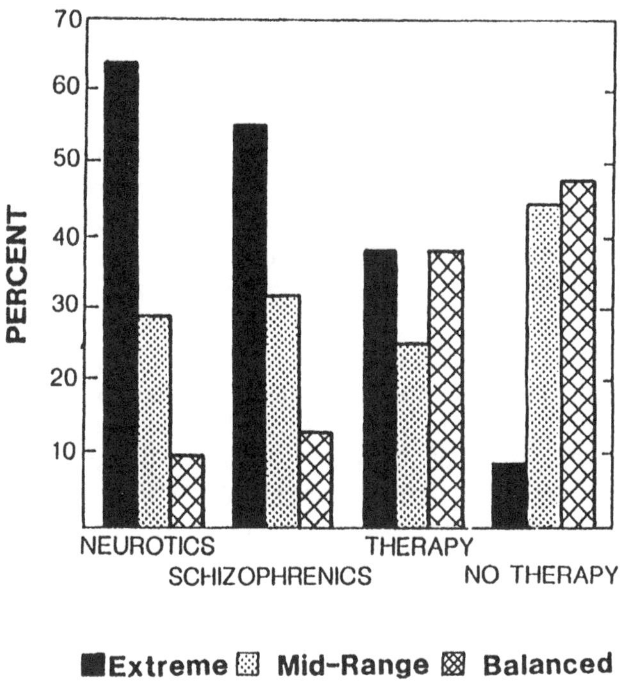

and schizophrenic groups compared to the no-therapy group. Conversely, he found a significantly higher level of balanced families in the no-therapy group compared to the other groups.

Figure 4 illustrates the differences in the levels of cohesion and adaptability between these groups. While the percentage of extreme family types decreased dramatically from the symptomatic to no-therapy groups (neurotic, 64%; schizophrenic, 56%; therapy, 38%; no therapy, 7%), the percentage of balanced families increased (neurotic, 8%; schizophrenic, 12%; therapy, 38%; no therapy, 48%) as hypothesized.

Other studies have focused on alcoholic families in which the identified patient was the mother or father. Using the original FACES, Olson and Killorin (1984) found significant differences between the chemically dependent families and the nondependent families. As hypothesized, alcoholic families had a significantly higher level of extreme families compared to the nondependent family. Over 20% of the chemically dependent families were extreme types, while only 4% of the nondependent families were extreme types. Conversely, about two-thirds (65%) of the nondependent families were balanced, while about one-third (38% and 32%) of the dependent families were balanced.

A study of alcoholics in treatment by Bonk (1984) assessed 20 families before treatment (pre), after treatment (post), and one month after treatment (follow-up). While no changes occurred over time on cohesion and adaptability, significant changes did occur between pre/post and pre/follow-up on the family satisfaction scale (27), which measures satisfaction on cohesion and adaptability.

A recent study by Carnes (1987) that used FACES II investigated the family systems in sex offenders and found high levels of extreme family types in both their family of origin and their current families (see Figure 5). While about half (49%) had extreme family types in their family of origin and about two-thirds (66%) of their current families were extreme types, only 19% of the nonoffender families were extreme. Conversely, while only 11% of their family of origin and 19% of their current families were balanced types, about half (57%) of the nonoffender families were balanced.

Comparing 27 high risk families with 35 low risk families, Garbarino, Sebes, and Schellenbach (1985) focused on the type of fam-

FIGURE 5: Sex Offenders

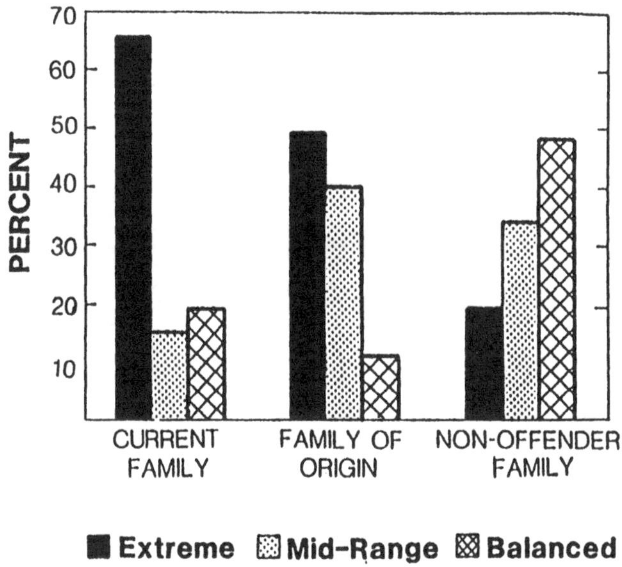

ily systems using FACES. Using intact families, both parents and one adolescent completed FACES and a variety of other scales that were used to assess family stress, parenting, and family conflict. As hypothesized by the Circumplex Model, they found the majority of the low risk families were balanced type (mainly flexibly connected) while the majority of the high risk families were an extreme type (mainly chaotically enmeshed).

A recent study by Rodick, Henggeler, and Hanson (1986) compared 58 mother-son dyads from father-absent families in which half (29) had an adolescent juvenile offender and the other half (29) had adolescents with no history of arrest or psychiatric referral. As graphically illustrated in Figure 6, only 7% of the delinquents were balanced while 93% of the delinquent families were mid-range or extreme types. In contrast, 69% of the nondelinquent families were balanced while 31% were mid-range or extreme.

In summary, these studies of clinical samples clearly demonstrate the discriminant power of the Circumplex Model in distinguishing

FIGURE 6: Delinquent Families

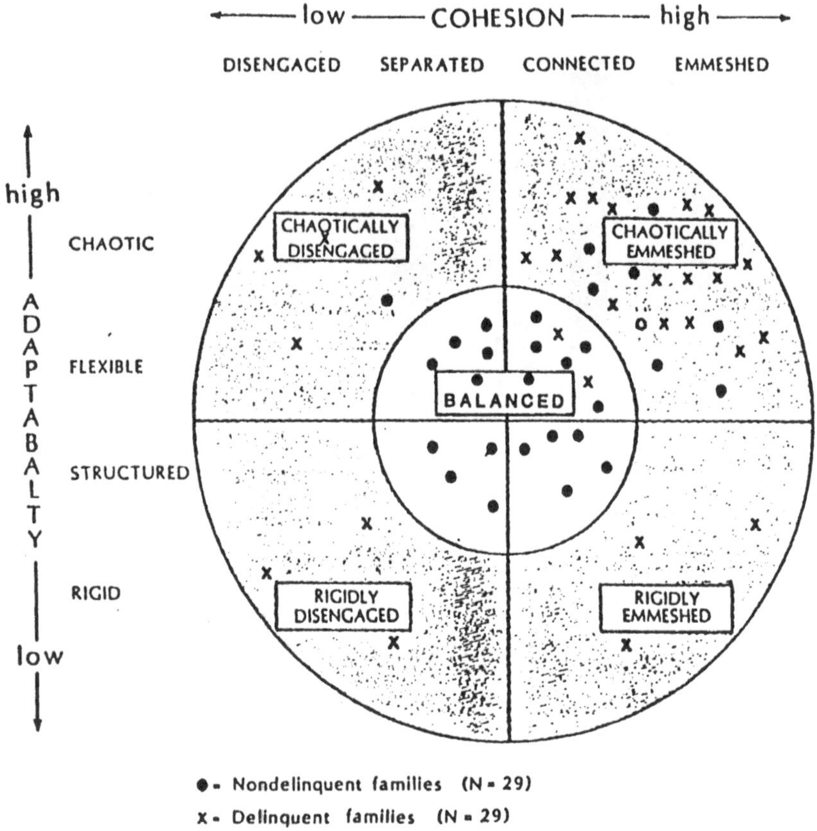

between problem families and nonsymptomatic families. There is strong empirical support for the hypothesis that balanced types of families are more function than extreme family types. There is, however, a lack of evidence that any of these symptoms are specifically linked with a specific type of family system, for example, chaotically enmeshed. This was the hope of early family research linking family symptoms (a schizophrenic offspring) and family systems.

In contrast to the curvilinear relationship found on these dimensions of problem families, there appears to be a linear relationship between cohesion and change (adaptability) in family functioning with "normal" families. More specifically, higher levels of cohesion and change seem to be associated with better family functioning. These results were found in the national survey with 1,000 families across the life cycle, which was reported in the recent book by Olson and colleagues, *Families: What Makes Them Work?* (1983). A primary reason for this finding is that normal families represent only a narrow spectrum of the range of behavior on these two dimensions. As a result, there are very few of the "normal" families that legitimately fall into the extreme types.

Balanced Families and Communication

Another hypothesis is that balanced families will have more positive communication skills than extreme families. Communication can be measured at both the marital and family level. Using data from the national survey of 1,000 families, Barnes and Olson (1982, 1983) investigated parent-adolescent communication and family functioning. Using "nonproblem" families, the hypothesis that balanced families would have better communication skills was supported when relying on data from the parents. However, this hypothesis was not supported for adolescents. Future research is needed to test hypotheses at both the marital and family level with both normal and problem families.

In addition to testing the hypothesis regarding balanced versus extreme families reviewed earlier, Rodick et al. (1986) found strong support for the hypothesis that balanced families have more positive communication skills. Using observational measures of mother-adolescent interaction, they found that mothers in the balanced group had significantly higher rates of supportive communication, explicit information, and positive affect than did the extreme type with the majority of problem dyads (chaotically enmeshed).

Accounting for Cultural and Ethnic Diversity Using Family Satisfaction

In order to make the Circumplex Model culturally relevant to a variety of families with different ethnic and cultural backgrounds, a hypothesis was developed to reflect this diversity. The hypothesis states that if normative expectations of families support behavior extreme on one or both of the dimensions, families will function well as long as all family members are satisfied with these expectations. In this way, the family serves as its own norm base.

This approach necessitates measuring family satisfaction of each family member. There have been two methods to measure family satisfaction related to the Circumplex Model. The first method is to have family members complete FACES III twice, once in terms of how they perceive their family system (perceived version) and second, for how they ideally would like it to be (ideal version). The greater the ideal-perceived discrepancy, the greater the dissatisfaction with the current family system.

The second method is a separate 14-item Family Satisfaction scale developed by Olson and Wilson (1982) that taps the concepts related to cohesion and change. A study by Caron and Olson (1984) identified, as hypothesized, a high negative correlation between family satisfaction scale and the ideal perceived discrepancy on cohesion ($r = -.58$) and on adaptability ($r = -.64$).

While it might be more difficult to observe change in cohesion and adaptability (and related family types) related to treatment, family satisfaction might be more sensitive to treatment change. This was demonstrated in a recent treatment outcome study of alcoholics by Bonk (1984). While he found no change in mean scores on cohesion or adaptability, significant increases in family satisfaction occurred between pre-post and pre-follow-up assessments.

INVENTORIES FOR CLINICAL ASSESSMENT AND RESEARCH

In order to adequately assess the three major dimensions of the Circumplex Model and other related concepts, Olson and colleagues (1982) have developed a variety of self-reports assessment tools. These assessment tools were designed to provide an "insider's perspective" on their own family system, but also an "outsider's perspective." The self-report instrument FACES III provides the insider's perspective, whereas the Clinical Rating Scale (CRS) provides the outsider's perspective. Both perspectives are useful and often provide conflicting data. Used together, however,

Olson discovered they help capture the complexity of marital and family systems (Olson, 1977).

FACES III: Self-Report Scale

FACES III, acronym for Family Adaptability and Cohesion Evaluation Scales, was developed by Olson, Portner and Lavee (1985) to tap cohesion and adaptability. FACES III provides an assessment of how an individual perceives their family system and also their ideal descriptions. The scores on cohesion and adaptability can be plotted onto the Circumplex Model to indicate the type of system they perceive and would like ideally. In addition, the perceived-ideal discrepancy also provides a measure of family satisfaction which indicates how satisfied individuals are with their current system regardless of their family type.

FACES III is a newly developed 20-item scale from items used in the national survey of 1,000 "normal" families (Olson et al., 1983). FACES III overcomes most of the limitation of FACES II which was also developed from the same sample. In FACES II, cohesion and adaptability were rather highly correlated with each other, with social desirability, and with marital and family satisfaction.

Ideally, the two dimensions in the Circumplex Model should be uncorrelated or orthogonal. Cohesion and adaptability in FACES III meets this criteria ($r = .03$). Because social desirability has an impact on most self-report scales, an attempt was made to minimize its impact on these two dimensions. In FACES III the correlation between adaptability and social desirability was reduced to zero ($r = .00$) with some correlation between social desirability and cohesion ($r = .39$).

FACES III is designed to measure both perceived and ideal descriptions of a marital or family system. The 20-item FACES III is taken twice, once for perceived and one for ideal description of the family. The perceived-ideal discrepancy is an indirect measure of family satisfaction. The greater the ideal-perceived discrepancy, the less the family satisfaction.

Family satisfaction is a very important variable which can be useful empirically and clinically. Empirically it provides an addition variable from FACES III for any analysis. Clinically, this information regarding both perceived and ideal is particularly useful. Whereas the perceived description can provide a perspective on the perception of the current system, the ideal can provide directions for change on both dimensions.

A summary evaluation of FACES III in terms of reliability, validity, and clinical utility is provided in Table 3. In general, FACES III is a reliable and valid scale that is theoretically based and is designed for systematic research or clinical work with couples and families. It was designed so that it could be used with a variety of family structures including nuclear families, blended families and single parent families.

For an illustration of a graphic representation of perceived and ideal FACES III scores from a father, mother and adolescent, see Figure 7. While the mother and father both perceived their family as a "structurally separated" type, the adolescent perceived the family as "rigidly enmeshed." Ideally, the parents both wanted more cohesion, but the mother wanted more adaptability and the father wanted less. However, the adolescent ideally wanted much less cohesion and more adaptability as characterized by the "flexibility disengaged" type. Viewing the ideal-perceived discrepancy, the adolescent is the least satisfied, as demonstrated by considerable perceived-ideal discrepancy. This graphic scheme clearly demonstrates the complexity of the family system in terms of how they perceive the family but also how they like their family to function.

Self-report instruments were also developed to measure both the marital communication and parent-adolescent communication. Marital communication can be assessed by a 10-item scale developed by Olson, Fournier, and Druckman (1986) from the ENRICH Inventory. Family communication was measured by the Parent-Adolescent Communication Scale (PAC) developed by Barnes and Olson (1985). This scale assesses two aspects of communication: open communication and problem-free communication. Parents describe how they perceive their communication with their adolescent and the adolescent describes the communication (1) with their father and (2) with their mother.

TABLE 3: EVALUATION OF FACES III

	FAMILY ADAPTABILITY & COHESION EVALUATION SCALE (FACES III)
Theoretical Domain and Model	Family System Circumplex Model
Assessment Level	Family as Whole
Focus of Assessment	Perceived, Ideal; Satisfaction
Number of Scales and Items	2 Scales; 20 perceived 20 ideal items
Norms	
Normative Sample	n = 2453 adults across life cycle n = 412 adolescents
Clinical	Several types of problem families
Reliability	
Internal Consistency	Cohesion (r = .77) Adaptability (r = .62) Total (r = .68)
Test Retest	FACES II (4-5 weeks) .83 for cohesion .80 for adaptability
Validity	
Face Valditiy	Very good evidence
Content Validity	Very good evidence
Correlation between Scales	Cohesion & Adaptability (r = .03)
Correlation with Social Desirability	SD & Adaptability (r = .00) SD & Cohesion (r = .39)
Concurrent Validity	Lack of evidence
Correlation between Family Members	X=H/W/A (n = 370) Cohesion (r = .41) Adaptability (r = .25)
Discrimination between Groups	Very good evidence
Clinical Utility	
Usefulness of Self-Report Scale	Very good evidence
Ease of Scoring	Easy
Clinical Rating Scale	Yes

FIGURE 7: Circumplex Model
Profile of Family

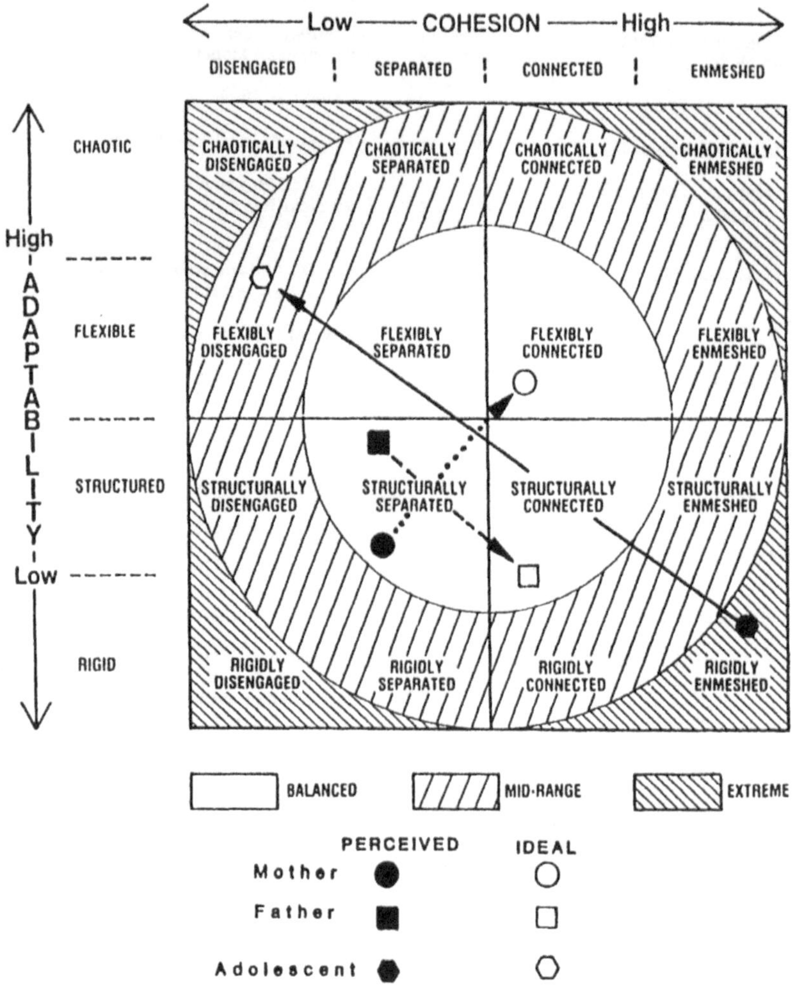

Clinical Rating Scale for the Circumplex Model

The Clinical Rating Scale (CRS) was developed by Olson and Killorin (1984) in order to do clinical assessment on cohesion, change and communication. The actual Clinical Rating Scale (CRS) is presented in Appendix A which illustrates the specific clinical indicators for each level of the three dimensions. This scale is a useful training device for helping therapists learn more about the Circumplex Model and its clinical usefulness (see Appendix A). Complete instructions for using and scoring the CRS can be obtained by writing the first author.

A Family Profile is used to summarize the ratings on these three dimensions. The CRS can be used for rating the behavior of a family system based on semi-structured interview with an individual family member or several members. Ideally, it is best to observe the family as they interact while completing some interaction tasks or during a semi-structured interview dealing with the concepts related to the three dimensions.

One useful format to generate information and dynamics about these dimensions is to ask the family member(s) to describe and discuss how they handle daily routines, what a typical weekend is like, and what they do separately and together and how they make decisions.

We have found the CRS easy for practitioners to learn and use in their clinical practice. Inter-rater reliability with this scale has been assessed at rather high levels (r = .70 – .80) in a recent study by Olson and Logacz (1985).

Clinical Assessment of a Chaotically Disengaged Family

Using the Clinical Rating Scale, the three dimensions of cohesion, change and communication are organized into eight-point scales. The Family Profile is used to summarize the global ratings on these three dimensions and the numerous concepts related for each of the dimensions. The ratings for the following family were based on the first semi-structured interview with them after they were referred for treatment.

The Kelly family was referred to a family therapist because of a court referral for physical abuse between the father, Harold, and the

14-year-old stepdaughter, Elaine. The mother, Margaret, also had experienced some physical abuse and had no other children. The final assessment was that the family was chaotically disengaged with very poor communication skills. The results of the clinical assessment are summarized on the Family Profile in Table 4.

On family cohesion, the global assessment for the family was a 2, indicating that they were a disengaged family. This global evaluation was based on their overall functioning after looking at the six major areas related to cohesion. More specifically, in regard to emotional bonding the family had extreme levels of emotional separateness and lacked family loyalty. In terms of family involvement, members had very little interaction with each other. Even though the affective responsiveness was infrequent, when it occurred it was often intense. The marital relationship was also characterized by extreme emotional separateness. Regarding parent-child coalitions, there was a lack of closeness between the father and daughter, but a rather strong closeness between the mother and adolescent. The internal boundaries were characterized by high separateness in that family members seldom spent time with each other and usually shared separate spaces in their home. Their external boundaries were mainly focused outside the family where they saw their separate friends and participated in separate interests and recreation. In conclusion, this family was rated very low across most of the concepts related to cohesion and could best be characterized as a "disengaged" family system (see Table 4).

In regard to family change (adaptability), the family generally functioned as a "chaotic" family system. Regarding leadership, neither the father nor the mother exercised much leadership in the family. The discipline of the daughter was often very lenient and the parents were inconsistent in their punishment. The negotiation regarding problems was often endless and while they agreed on decisions, they rarely carried them out. The roles in the household were characterized by a great deal of role ambiguity, since no one felt responsible for taking care of the most routine responsibilities. The family rules frequently changed and were inconsistently enforced. As a result, the Kelly family tended to function as a "chaotic" family system (see Table 4).

The family communication was generally very poor and it did not

TABLE 4: FAMILY PROFILE OF A CHAOTICALLY DISENGAGED FAMILY

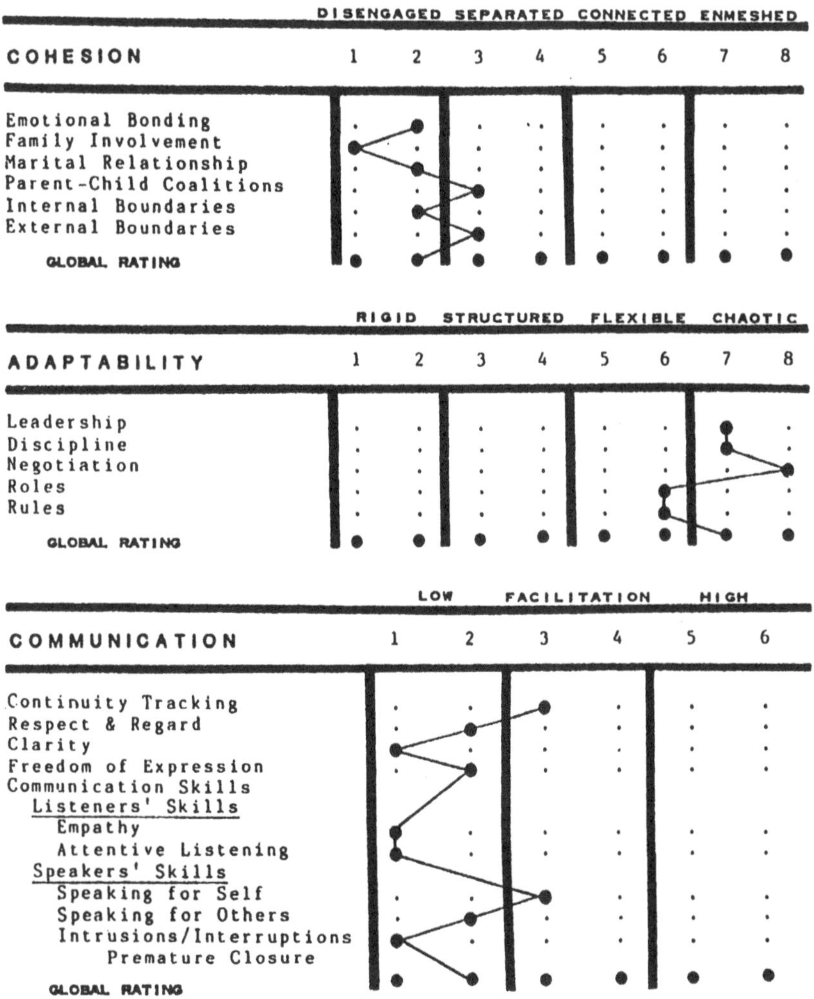

facilitate understanding or movement on either cohesion or adaptability dimensions. After observing their family interaction, it was apparent that their continuity of tracking was generally good but sometimes was inconsistent in that members would make distracting nonverbal asides. There was little respect and regard for each other. The clarity of their communication was problematic because they often made incongruent and at times double binding messages. Their freedom of expression was low but at times they were willing to express negative feelings but not positive ones about each other. In general, their listening skills were very poor in that they had low levels of empathy and attentive listening. Their speaking skills were sometimes good in that they were willing to assert themselves but they also made frequent interruptions when others were taking. In conclusion, their communication skills were generally poor as a family system.

REFERENCES

Barnes, H., & Olson, D. H. (1982). Parent Adolescent Communication Scale. In D. Olson, H. I. McCubbin, H. Barnes, A. Larsen, M. Muxen, & M. Wilson (eds.), *Family inventories*. St. Paul, MN: Family Social Science, University of Minnesota.

Barnes, H., & Olson, D. H. (1983). Parent adolescent communication and the Circumplex Model. *Child Development, 56*, 438-447.

Beavers, W. R., & Voeller, M. N. (1983). Family models: Comparing and contrasting the Olson Circumplex Model and the Beavers Systems Model. *Family Process, 22*, 250-260.

Benjamin, Lorna S. (1977). Structural analysis of a family in therapy. *J. Counsel. Clin. Psychol., 45*, 391-406.

Bonk, J. (1984). Perceptions of psychodynamics during a transitional period as reported by families affected by alcoholism. Unpublished doctoral dissertation, University of Arizona.

Carnes, P. (1987). *Counseling sexual abusers*. Minneapolis: CompCare Publications.

Caron, W., & Olson, D. H. (1984). *Family satisfaction and perceived-ideal discrepancy on FACES II*. St. Paul, MN: Family Social Science, University of Minnesota.

Clarke, J. (1984). The family types of schizophrenics, neurotics and "normals." Unpublished doctoral dissertation, Family Social Science, University of Minnesota.

Constantine, L. (1986). *Family paradigms*. New York: Guilford Press.

Epstein, N. B., Bishop, D. S., & Lewis, S. (1978). The McMaster Model of family functioning. *Journal of Marriage and Family Counseling*, *4*, 19-31.

French, A. P., & Guidera, B. J. (1974). The family as a system in four dimensions: A theoretical model. Paper presented at the American Academy of Child Psychology, San Francisco, CA.

Garbarino, J., Sebes, J., & Schellenbach, C. (1985). Families at risk for destructive parent-child relations in adolescents. *Child Development*, *55*, 174-183.

Gaughan, L. D. (1982). Structural theory of family mediation. In L. Messinger (ed.), *Therapy with remarriage families*. Rockville: Aspen System Corporation.

Gottman, J. M. (1979). *Marital interaction*. New York: Basic Books.

Hill, R. (1970). *Family development in three generations*. Cambridge, MA: Schenkman.

Kantor, D., & Lehr (1975). *Inside the family*. San Francisco: Jossey-Bass.

L'Abate, L. (1985). The emperor has no clothes! Long live the emperor! A critique of family systems thinking and a reductionist proposal. Unpublished manuscript.

Leary, T. (1957). *Interpersonal diagnosis of personality*. New York: Ronald Press.

Leff, J., & Vaughn, C. (1985). *Expressed emotion in families*. New York: Guilford Press.

Olson, D. H. (1977). Insiders' and outsiders' view of relationships: Research strategies. In G. Levinger and H. Rausch (eds.), *Close relationships*. Amherst, MA: University of Massachusetts Press.

Olson, D. H., Fournier, D. G., & Druckman, J. M. (1986). *PREPARE, PREPARE-MC & ENRICH Inventories*. Minneapolis: PREPARE/ENRICH, Inc., P. O. Box 190, Minneapolis, MN 55458.

Olson, D. H., & Killorin, E. (1984). *Clinical Rating Scale for Circumplex Model*. St. Paul, MN: Family Social Science, University of Minnesota, Revised Version.

Olson, D. H., McCubbin, H. I., Barnes, H., Larsen, A., Muxen, M., & Wilson, M. (1983). *Family inventories*. St. Paul, MN: Family Social Science, University of Minnesota.

Olson, D. H., McCubbin, H. I., Barnes, H., Larsen, A., Muxen, M., & Wilson, M. (1983). *Families: What makes them work*. Los Angeles: Sage Publishing.

Olson, D. H., Portner, J., & Lavee, Y. (1985). *FACES III*. St. Paul, MN: Family Social Science, University of Minnesota.

Olson, D. H., Russell, C. S., & Sprenkle, D. H. (1983). Circumplex Model VI: Theoretical update. *Family Process*, *22*, 69-83.

Olson, D. H., & Wilson, M. (1982). Family satisfaction. In D. Olson et al. (eds.), *Family inventories*. St. Paul, MN: Family Social Science, University of Minnesota.

Olson, D. H. (1986). Circumplex Model VII: Validation studies and FACES III. *Family Process*, *25*, 337-351.

Parsons, T., & Bales, R. F. (1955). *Family socialization and interaction process*. Glencoe, IL: Free Press.

Reiss, D. (1981). *The family's construction of reality*. Cambridge: Harvard University Press.

Rodick, J. D., Henggler, S. W., & Hanson, C. L. (1986). An evaluation of Family Adaptability and Cohesion Evaluation Scales (FACES) and the Circumplex Model. *Journal of Abnormal Child Psychology*, *14*, 77-87.

Appendix A: Clinical Rating Scale - Family Cohesion

	COUPLE/ FAMILY SCORE	DISENGAGED (Very Low) 1 2	SEPARATED (Low to Moderate) 3 4	CONNECTED (Moderate to High) 5 6	ENMESHED (Very High) 7 8
EMOTIONAL BONDING		Extreme emotional separateness. Lack of family loyalty.	Emotional separateness. Occasional family loyalty.	Emotional closeness. Loyalty to family expected.	Extreme emotional closeness. Loyalty to family is demanded.
FAMILY INVOLVEMENT		Very low involvement or interaction between members. Infrequent affective responsiveness between members.	Involvement acceptable but personal distance preferred. Some affective responsiveness is demonstrated.	Involvement emphasized but personal distance allowed. Affective interactions encouraged and preferred.	Very high symbiotic involvement, members very dependent on each oth[er]. Affective dependency is demonstrate[d].
MARITAL RELATIONSHIP		Extreme emotional separateness.	Emotional separateness.	Emotional closeness.	Extreme emotional reactivity.
PARENT-CHILD COALITIONS		Lack of parent-child closeness.	Clear sub-system boundaries some p/c closeness.	Clear sub-system boundaries with parent-child closeness.	Parent-child coalition. Lack of generational boundaries.
INTERNAL BOUNDARIES		Personal separateness predominant.	Some personal separateness encouraged.	Need for separateness respected but less valued.	Lack of personal separateness.
TIME (physical & emotional)		Time apart from family maximized. Rarely time together.	Time alone important. Some time together.	Time together important. Time alone permitted.	Time together maximized. Little time alone permitted.
SPACE (physical & emotional)		Separate space needed and preferred.	Separate space preferred; sharing of family space.	Sharing family space. Private space respected.	Little private space permitted.
DECISION MAKING		Independent decision making.	Individual decision making but joint possible.	Joint decisions preferred but not necessary.	Decisions subject to wishes of entire group.

Appendix A (continued): Clinical Rating Scale - Family Cohesion

	COUPLE/ FAMILY SCORE	DISENGAGED (Very Low) 1 2	SEPARATED (Low to Moderate) 3 4	CONNECTED (Moderate to High) 5 6	ENMESHED (Very High) 7 8
EMOTIONAL BONDING		Extreme emotional separateness. Lack of family loyalty.	Emotional separateness. Occasional family loyalty.	Emotional closeness. Loyalty to family expected.	Extreme emotional closeness. Loyalty to family is demanded.
EXTERNAL BOUNDARIES		Mainly focused outside the family.	More focused outside than inside family.	More focused inside than outside family.	Mainly focused inside the family.
FRIENDS		Individual friends seen alone.	Individual friendships seldom shared with family.	Individual friendships shared with family.	Family friends preferred with limited individual friends.
INTERESTS		Disparate interests.	Separate interests.	Joint interests preferred.	Joint interests mandated.
RECREATION		Mainly separate recreation.	More separate than shared. recreation.	More shared than individual recreation.	
GLOBAL COHESION RATING (1-8)					

Appendix A (continued)

Appendix A: Clinical Rating Scale - Family Adaptability

	COUPLE OR FAMILY SCORE	RIGID (Very Low) 1 2	STRUCTURED (Low to Moderate) 3 4	FLEXIBLE (Moderate to High) 5 6	CHAOTIC (Very High) 7 8
LEADERSHIP (Control)		Authoritarian leadership. Parent(s) highly controlling.	Primarily authoritarian but some equalitarian leadership.	Equalitarian leadership with fluid changes.	Limited and/or erratic leadership. Parental control unsuccessful, rebuffed.
DISCIPLINE (For Families Only)		Autocratic, "law & order". Strict, rigid consequences. Not lenient.	Somewhat democratic. Predictable consequences. Seldom lenient.	Usually democratic. Negotiated consequences. Somwhat lenient.	Laissez-faire and ineffective. Inconsistent consequences. Very lenient.
NEGOTIATION		Limited negotiations. Decisions imposed by parents	Structured negotiations. Decisions mainly made by parents.	Flexible negotiations. Agreed upon decisions.	Endless negotiations. Impulsive decisions.
ROLES		Limited repertoire; strictly defined roles.	Roles stable, but may be shared.	Role sharing and making. Fluid changes of roles.	Lack of role clarity, role shifts and role reversals.
RULES		Unchanging rules. Rules strictly enforced.	Few rule changes. Rules firmly enforced	Some rule changes. Rules flexibly enforced.	Frequent rule changes. Rules inconsistently enforced.
GLOBAL ADAPTABILITY RATING (1-8)					

Appendix A (continued)

Appendix A: Clinical Rating Scale - Family Communication

	COUPLE OR FAMILY SCORE	LOW ---------FACILITATING--------- HIGH 1–2	3–4	5–6
CONTINUITY TRACKING		Little continuity of content; Irrelevant/distracting non-verbals and asides frequently occur; Frequent/inappropriate topic changes;	Some continuity but not consistent across time or across all members; Some irrelevant/distracting non-verbals and asides; Topic changes not consistently appropriate;	Members consistently tracking; Few irrelevant/distracting non-verbals and asides; facilitative non-verbals; Appropriate topic changes;
RESPECT & REGARD		Lack of respect for feelings or message of other(s); possibly overtly disrespectful or belittling attitude;	Somewhat respectful of others but not consistent across time or across all members;	Consistently appears respectful of others' feelings and message;
CLARITY		Inconsistent and/or unclear verbal messages; Frequent incongruencies between verbal and non-verbal messages;	Some degree of clarity; but not consistent across time or across all members; Some incongruent messages;	Verbal messages very clear. Generally congruent messages;
FREEDOM OF EXPRESSION		Infrequent discussion of self, feelings and relationships;	Some discussion of self, feelings and relationships;	Open discussion of self, feelings and relationships;
COMMUNICATION SKILL				
Listeners' Skills				
Empathy		Seldom evident	Sometimes evident	Often evident
Attentive Listening		Seldom evident	Sometimes evident	Often evident
Speakers' Skills				
Speaking for Self		Seldom evident	Sometimes evident	Often evident
Speaking for Others		Often evident	Sometimes evident	Seldom evident
Intrusions/Interruptions Premature Closure		Often evident	Sometimes evident	Seldom evident
GLOBAL FAMILY COMMUNICATION RATING (1-6)				

Building Relationship Skills in Families and Para-Family Teams

Bernard Guerney, Jr.
Louise Guerney

ABSTRACT. The use of family members as psychotherapeutic agents for one another represents a largely untapped, very powerful source for helping children and youth. At a time of scarce financial resources, it would be especially regrettable not to use it. A skill-training approach is viewed as an especially useful strategy for harnessing family-power. An example of such an approach, Relationship Enhancement is presented and its actual and potential uses are described.

The number of individuals in social or psychological trouble is increasing. The funds available for helping them are decreasing. Mental health professionals and paraprofessionals owe it to themselves and to their clients to seek innovative means of helping. They should explore new, inexpensive sources of manpower to assist them in the helping process. One such source—family members—offers something far more than just inexpensive labor. Family members often offer a means of helping that is far more powerful than professional or para-professional helpers could hope to provide on their own.

No paid team of helpers is likely to hold stronger power—whether for good or bad—to influence a troubled, dysfunctional person than members of his or her family. The trick is to turn that enormous power from one which is destructive, inoperative, or just moderately positive to one which is strongly positive. When that

Bernard Guerney, Jr. and Louise Guerney are affiliated with the Family Consultation Center, College of Health and Human Development, Pennsylvania State University, University Park, PA 16802.

objective is accomplished, it is the equivalent of getting, at no cost, co-workers who are exceptionally effective. The same is true when a mental health worker enlists the aid of those whom we'd call "para-family" members. By para-family members we mean foster parents, parent surrogates in residential treatment settings, or special community-based homes and halfway houses, or even co-residents in such settings.

To become consistently effective in recruiting and empowering family or para-family members as helpers, we believe most mental health workers will need to acquire new attitudes and methods. The new attitudes are much more difficult to acquire than the new methods, because they are quite a radical departure from tradition.

THE EDUCATIONAL MODEL

Relationship enhancement is a conceptual model which is well-suited to helping individuals overcome psychosocial problems and to enlisting the aid of family members in the process. It is an educational or skill-building model (Authier, Gustafson, B. Guerney, & Kasdorf, 1975; B. Guerney, 1977, 1982; B. Guerney, L. Guerney, & Stollak, 1971/1972; B. Guerney, Stollak, & L. Guerney, 1970, 1971). In this model, the clients' psychosocial problems are viewed as the result of ordinary learning processes (including learning to use denial and other defense mechanisms) and/or the failure to learn appropriate psychosocial skills. Solutions are viewed as stemming from new learning. Instead of being based on the physician's approach to helping, the approach is based on the teacher's way of learning.

The way clients are approached in the educational model is in striking contrast to the medical model. Although only "clients" are mentioned, the same thing applies equally to family members recruited as helpers. In the educational, skill-building model, the concept that the clients have unfulfilled ambitions replaces the concept that clients are sick. The client is much like us and is to be related to in the same manner as we would wish to be. The need for helping clients to *clarify and set their own goals*, with an awareness of the demands which society and other people will make upon them, replaces the need to diagnose.

Designing an appropriate systematic skill or choosing an already existing psychosocial skill *training program* replaces the *prescriptive* process in which a unique program is designed for each client in accord with the client's experiences. The relationship factors and therapeutic methods are arranged in such a way as to effect the changes chosen by the helper.

The concept of contracting with informed clients to *teach* them clearly specified skills replaces the concept of *treatment* wherein the clients usually are not aware of what they are supposed to be learning, if anything, from their interactions with the helper. The concept of eliminating problems in the course of seeking positive objectives through the *additive* process of learning concepts and skills which the average person does not have, to *fulfill ambitions and achieve goals*, replaces the *subtractive* process of cure which seeks to restore a condition of "normalcy." This model eliminates many of the difficulties the service provider and the clients face when the guiding strategy for helping is based on analogies with medical practices.

The question often is raised, does this model work when the clients are seemingly unaware that they have problems or are "unmotivated"—e.g., court referred cases say for spouse-battering or alcoholism. The answer is that it seems to be even *more* useful in such instances.

Physicians deal mainly with people who are afraid for themselves and in pain. They are, therefore, usually willing to do whatever the physician tells them to do. Also, the results which physicians' prescriptions achieve are very often easy to foresee and fairly immediate. Possibly because of this, physicians have concerned themselves little with how to motivate their patients. When a patient fails to follow a prescription, well that's the patient's fault.

Consequently, psychosocial service providers who follow the medical model likewise frequently do not regard a failure to motivate clients as a failure of treatment per se. Instead, the unmotivated clients are viewed as responsible for the failure, and given labels ("character disorder," "sociopath," "narcissist," and the like). It is the patient who is responsible for either not undertaking, dropping out of, or failing in the therapy.

In the educational model, the teacher deals with results that require considerable and prolonged effort. The payoff for the skills learned usually is neither immediate nor easily foreseeable by the student. Therefore, motivating the student is considered an integral part of the teacher's responsibilities. "Motivated" is a state teachers assume they often will have to *create* and work continuously to maintain; it is not viewed as something the student brings as an initial characteristic. Thus, therapists following the educational model regard doing the things necessary to motivate clients and keep them motivated as the first and foremost aspects of their job.

Motivating the Client

What motivating the client means in the educational model is that the therapist must match what he or she will teach with the goals that the client and the family members want to achieve. For example, spouse abusers, who almost never consciously wish to beat their wives, must be brought to see that they can both eliminate that behavior and better achieve their most important goals by learning certain skills. Alcoholics must be made to see that the goals they are foregoing by continuing to drink may really be more important to them than those met by drinking. They also must be brought to see that it is possible for them to achieve the goals they do achieve by drinking—usually *feelings* such as competence, reduced anxiety, and lowered inhibition—through the acquisition of pertinent skills rather than through the illusory and short-lived method of alcohol consumption.

Once motivation is kindled (or more accurately, once the participants can perceive that the therapist can help them achieve the goals they were motivated to achieve all along), the teaching therapy can begin. Through the therapist's encouragement and the client's successes, the motivation not only can be maintained, but it is likely to grow stronger over the course of therapy. Using the educational model, the batterer's or alcoholic's wife and/or other family members can be more readily recruited to become an aide to the service provider. From there, one proceeds to changing the family system—through the skill-training process.

Some major barriers to kindling the motivation of family members to be of help to clients are eliminated in the educational model.

These barriers, which are difficult to erase in other approaches, are based on fear and ignorance. Fear occurs because they assume the therapist will seek to demonstrate the weaknesses of the family members or seek to change their personalities or self-image.

The Recruitment of Family Members

Detailed suggestions on recruiting and working with parents of young children and adolescents by using an educational model may be found elsewhere (B. Guerney, L. Guerney, & Stover, 1972; Vogelsong & B. Guerney, 1980). The general point is that once a mental health service provider is willing to try the positive approach of skill-building, many of the presumed or real difficulties in enlisting and maintaining the aid of family members in the treatment process fall away. The family members come to be seen not as enemies who themselves must first be treated before they can be trusted, but instead as allies, as teammates in the treatment process.

Family members can be viewed from the start as psychotherapeutic agents (B. Guerney, 1969) enlisted by the therapist to help the client. They are not being asked to expose their dynamics, thoughts, or feelings to the analysis of the mental health worker before they can begin to help. When such exposure occurs later as an integral part of the helping process, they have much less fear of such exposure.

The motivation of the family members in this model is not that of changing their own "pathology," or "pathology-inducing" behavior, in order to help the client. Rather, they are being asked to acquire new skills. It is important that they understand that such skills are not those which other ordinary people have. Rather, they are rare skills which previously only mental health workers possessed, and which are now to be taught to *them*. They are not being asked to give up their weaknesses or to become more normal, they are being permitted to acquire skills which normal people do *not* have.

Family members are not being asked to give up anything, but to acquire skills which they can choose to make use of in any given set of circumstances. Moreover, these skills will be useful to them not only in permitting them to better help the client, but in achieving their own family goals. Most family members are not only willing, but eager to take advantage of such an opportunity. Because of the absence of threat and the promise of special expertise, "resistance" usually is nil, and enthusiasm for participating is frequently high.

Specific Helping Skills and Methods of Relationship Enhancement (RE)

What are the various skills which clients and family members can learn in order to overcome their problems through achieving their goals, and what systematic program exists for teaching those skills? Today, there are many skill-building approaches for use with clients or families which the interested service-provider should explore (Larson, 1984; Marshall & Kurtz, 1982).

To illustrate the use of a skill-training approach to enlisting the aid of family members in the treatment process, we will concentrate on one set of programs: *Relationship Enhancement (RE) programs*. RE is chosen for a number of reasons. One is that we know it best. Another is that its effectiveness has been well demonstrated through controlled research (Collins, 1977; D'Augelli, Deyss, B. Guerney, Hershenberg, & Sborofsky, 1974; Ely, B. Guerney, & Stover, 1973; Ginsberg, 1977; Ginsberg & Vogelsong, 1977; Rappaport, 1976; Sywulak, 1977).

RE seems to be more powerful than other approaches in effecting improvement in family and para-family relationships (Brock & Joanning, 1983; Brown, 1980; Giblin, Sprenkle, & Sheehan, 1985; B. Guerney, Coufal, & Vogelsong, 1981; Jessee & B. Guerney, 1981; Ross, Baker, & B. Guerney, 1984). It has long lasting effects (Avery, Ridley, Leslie, & Milholland, 1980; B. Guerney, Vogelsong, & Coufal, 1983; L. Guerney, & Wolfgang, 1981; Sensue, 1981; Wieman, 1973). It can be taught with *relative* ease (L. Guerney, 1976a; Most & B. Guerney, 1983) because it is systematic, and because teaching aids are available both for therapists (Figley & B. Guerney, 1976; B. Guerney, 1985; L. Guerney, 1974, 1976b, in press; Vogelsong & B. Guerney, 1978, 1979), clients, and family members (B. Guerney, in press; B. Guerney & Vogelsong, 1981; L. Guerney, 1973, 1975, 1978).

The skills taught in an RE program are pertinent, often central, to most of the psychosocial problems which clients have. It is a program for achieving goals to which almost all of the subcultures within our society subscribe and, therefore, will be perceived as desirable by almost all clients and their family members. These overall goals, for both client and family members, are designed to achieve a sense of closeness, equity, and harmony with significant others. It is also designed to be able to derive support and help from family members in working through personal and interpersonal problems and conflicts.

In working with young children (under 12), the method used is Child or Filial RE (B. Guerney, 1983). In Child RE, the children who are the central beneficiaries of the program are not themselves trained in skills. Rather, the parents are trained in relationship and child management skills. The main vehicle used to train the parents in relationship and child management skills is play-therapy. The parents are taught to use their skills both at the mental health facility and, for nonresidential cases, at home. The parents then learn to transfer the attitudes and skills into their daily lives at home. Where play sessions are not feasible, the parents may be taught similar attitudes and behaviors through demonstration and role plays without the child being present.

With adolescents and older family members, all family members are treated alike and trained in the same RE skills (B. Guerney, 1977, 1984). The goals which the skills are designed to accomplish are: (1) Expressiveness—understanding of one's feelings and wishes in interpersonal relationships and a willingness to speak out about them to intimates in an honest and easily understood yet compassionate way; (2) Empathy—the ability to develop caring, understanding, and an appreciation of the ideas, feelings, and wishes of those with whom one wishes to develop or to deepen a close relationship; (3) Negotiation—the ability to carry on discussions and negotiations with others in such a way as to reveal the basic ideas, feelings, and wishes of all concerned; (4) Conflict Resolution—the ability to creatively develop realistic, long lasting, solutions to interpersonal conflicts and problems; (5) Self Changing—the ability to change one's way of thinking and behaving in consciously chosen ways; (6) Other Changing—the ability to help intimates to make such changes; (7) Generalization—the ability to put the above-mentioned capacities to work in a variety of settings and circumstances with a wide variety of people; (8) Teaching—the ability to help intimates to do likewise; and (9) Maintenance—the ability to permanently maintain the use of these capacities.

Participants: Family and Para-family

It is desirable to include all the members of a family or para-family who can be convinced to directly participate. Only those who would fail to learn the skills and also seriously disrupt the learning process for all the other participants are excluded (e.g., psychotic). The entire family, a sub-group in the family, or a single person may participate. When the entire relevant family group participates, it is called "omnilateral" RE. When a sub-group participates, it is called "multilateral" RE. When one individual participates, it is called "unilateral" RE. The focus of each of these types is not on the individual as such, but on improving the individuals' relationships with others, including those not present in the session.

RE focuses on the *system* as a whole; that is, on attaining the sought-after skillful patterns of *interaction* necessary to achieve the process and outcome goals. Generally, the problems of all family members are treated in an equitable manner. In many cases, such equity means a concentration of more time and attention on some members than others—frequently but not always, the targeted client. This occurs when the central person, the others, and the therapist all believe that such concentration best achieves the process and outcome goals of all family members. Relevant family members who are not physically present in the session are nevertheless always fully represented through a role-playing process.

Relationship improvement with nonpresent pertinent family members is accomplished in the following manner. As skills are learned, goals are established for improving the participants' relationships with other persons in the family. The use of the skills to accomplish such objectives is planned, then rehearsed, with the missing party or parties represented in role-playing. The participant then executes the plan in real life, and reports back on the usage of the skills and the outcome of the interaction. The person then receives appropriate reinforcement and feedback on skill usage.

Thus, RE remains a systems method even when only one member of a family participates. By virtue of the method just described, it remains a quite direct method for helping a target-client, even when he or she does *not* participate in the sessions. Conversely, the family members become helpers even when the target-client is the *only* one to participate in the sessions. This is the case because participants in RE learn how to elicit help and support from intimates who are not present in the sessions. A target participant whose family members are not present plans, rehearses, implements plans for getting help, and is given feedback on that process. It should also be pointed out in this connection that para-family members may include peers—e.g., fellow inpatients or residents, instead of or in addition to real family members.

Variety of Training Formats

The training of participants to secure and to provide help from others in a family or para-family may take place in a variety of formats in RE. As was earlier stated, the approach may be used with an individual, a sub-group of a family, or all family members. It may be used with a group of sole members of families, a group of sub-groups of families, or a group of families. Very experienced leaders sometimes work with larger numbers. Generally speaking, groups should be limited to no more than eight participants, preferably six.

With respect to time, sessions may be run in an *extended* format (45 to 90 minute sessions once or twice a week), or an *intensive* format. Three types of intensive formats are used. In a *marathon* format, sessions may last from three hours to a full day, usually repeated weekly (a common format is two consecutive days on a single weekend). *Mini-marathon* sessions run from one and one-half to three hours, usually repeated weekly. A *front-loaded* format is one which combines one or two mini-marathon sessions with extended sessions.

In RE skill training programs, it is desirable that the basic skills first be taught while discussing emotionally comfortable issues. Therefore, the front-loaded format has the advantage of cutting down the delay before clients can work on emotionally significant areas: they can work on emotionally "hot" issues during the first or second week of the program instead of the second or third. At the same time, because of the extended portion of the format, it provides opportunity for home assignments and skill-practice to go on between sessions. This provides economy and promotes transfer and generalization of skills. The weekend format is especially useful when the staff is being trained to coordinate the RE program.

In general, the various formats allow each agency to conduct RE in terms of its own possibilities and constraints. For example, a community-centered agency would probably find it most efficient and effective to follow an extended or front-loaded format. A residential setting serving a widely dispersed area, with family members visiting infrequently, might wish to hold mini-marathon or even marathon sessions. If a residential institution wishes to use its own staff and clients as an RE para-family, an extended format would probably serve best.

RE groups can be open-ended, with new members joining ongoing groups. In such circumstances, it is desirable to conduct a mini-marathon session for the newcomers *alone* to give them training in basic skills before they enter the group.

Leadership Training Requirements

Appropriate reading and audiovisual training materials and a weekend or preferably a three-day training program generally provide sufficient training to get a staff member or a staff ready to start an RE program in their setting. It is highly desirable to submit audio- or videotapes of the therapist at work for supervision by long-distance phone or return audiotape. One-day advanced workshops also are available for special problems and for supervision. Such training and (certification) is available nationally through a nonprofit institute.

Use in a Variety of Treatment Settings

Skill-training approaches in general, and RE in particular, may be used in virtually any setting. Participation of family members in the treatment process is not as difficult as most service providers probably believe. We will first consider *outpatient settings*. It is true that in lower-class communities parents are under so much pressure merely to survive that their recruitment as therapeutic assistants or agents may be difficult or impossible. It also is true that many lower middle-class single-parents are under so much time pressure that recruiting them and holding them is difficult. Nevertheless, there are fair numbers in both categories who show impressive and gratifying strength and determination in taking on this task. The agencies willing to provide a babysitter at the agency—for example during the time when a group of parents meets for Filial Therapy sessions—and helping one way or another in arranging transportation, can make a big difference. It is often feasible to secure the help of agency volunteers to implement this kind of assistance.

In *residential settings*, even when the children do not have the mental ability or sufficient reality contact to learn the skills themselves, it may be possible to recruit and train their parents (Vogelsong, B. Guerney, & L. Guerney, 1983). And even where parents cannot be involved, it should still be possible to give RE training to those staff members who have the most intimate contacts with the residents. They can then act as para-family therapeutic agents, using the skills regularly in their day-to-day contacts with the children.

In residential settings where parents cannot be recruited, but the children are generally over 12 years or so in mental age, it is possible to train *both* the children and those staff members who are in daily and frequent interaction with the children. They can then interact as a skills para-family. If desired, such interaction could come to involve not only the exploration of feelings and relationships, but the rules of behavior and discipline governing the para-family unit. This would be analogous to the "quality circles" used in business and industry settings.

Behavioral rehearsal for working through problems with their family on their home visits or after their permanent return to the family also could be a major feature of these para-family sessions, thereby combining a para-family and a family helping function in one group. Newcomers to both staff and resident population can learn the skills from the group through separate mini-marathon instruction and, mainly, by seeing them in use by the group.

In residential settings, it may be possible to request that family members plan regular visits of an hour and a half or more. If the visit is coordinated with a mental health worker's schedule, the worker can train, and later supervise, the family members' skilled interactions. The goal would be to improve their relationships and to provide emotional support to the target child and to one another. In some residential settings, it may be possible for parents to come in for a full day or more of training and of supervised use of the skills. This might be done during a weekend, or in conjunction with admission and/or termination procedures.

After discharge, a couple of mini-marathon sessions on a monthly basis would be a desirable feature for residential settings. This would be especially true when the family had not been regularly involved during the inpatient period.

Skill-training and RE programs involving family as psychotherapeutic agents are also appropriate for other types of settings. A few examples should suffice to demonstrate this. Many foster children are emotionally disturbed to one degree or another. RE-based programs training foster parents in RE skills pertinent both to younger children and adolescents have been conducted throughout the state of Pennsylvania, and in many other states (L. Guerney, 1976a, 1977). Studies showed that they were able to learn and retain the skills and considered them very useful (B. Guerney, Vogelsong, & Wolfgang, 1977; B. Guerney, Wolfgang, & Vogelsong, 1978; L. Guerney & Wolfgang, 1981).

Parole officers in a special unit were trained to train juvenile delinquents, their parents, and sometimes siblings, in RE skills. The families they worked with showed much improvement in their relationships (B. Guerney, Vogelsong, & Glynn, 1977). Staff of a community-based home for retarded children have been trained in RE methods. They found it a very valuable asset to themselves and the residents (Sywulak, 1984).

Workers in spouse abuse centers/shelters have trained not only the couples involved in RE skills to very good effect, but also trained battered mothers in Child RE principles. Clinical observations at our own facility and elsewhere indicate that Filial RE seems to be an effective approach for child abuse.

In a Drug and Alcohol Counseling Center, intimates (mostly

mates, but occasionally adolescent children) of alcoholics as well as the alcoholics themselves have been trained in RE skills. The program seemed to be very effective in maintaining abstinence (Matter, McAllister, & B. Guerney, 1984).

These examples of the uses to which RE has been put are intended to stimulate the reader's imagination toward using RE and other family and para-family skill-training methods to help clients in their own settings. The payoff, we believe, will be more than worth whatever attitudinal and procedural difficulties may be encountered. Harnessing the power of the family can, we believe, significantly improve the treatment effectiveness of virtually any child or adolescent service facility.

REFERENCES

Authier, J., Gustafson, K., Guerney, B., Jr., & Kasdorf, J. (1975). The psychological practitioner as a teacher: A theoretical-historical and practical review. *The Counseling Psychologist*, *5*(2), 31-50.

Avery, A. W., Ridley, C. A., Leslie, L. A., & Milholland, T. (1980). Relationship enhancement with premarital dyads: A six-month follow-up. *American Journal of Family Therapy*, *8*, 23-30.

Brock, G. W., & Joanning, H. (1983). A comparison of the relationship enhancement program and the Minnesota couple communication program. *Journal of Marital and Family Therapy*, *9*(4), 413-421.

Brown, D. L. (1980). *A comparative study of the effects of two foster parent training methods on attitudes of parental acceptance, sensitivity to children, and general foster parent attitudes*. Unpublished doctoral dissertation, Michigan State University.

Collins, J. D. (1977). Experimental evaluation of a six month conjugal therapy program. In B. Guerney, Jr. (Ed.), *Relationship enhancement: Skill training programs for therapy, problem prevention, and enrichment*. San Francisco: Jossey-Bass.

D'Augelli, A. R., Deyss, C. S., Guerney, B. G., Jr., Hershenberg, B., & Sborofsky, S. L. (1974). Interpersonal skill training for dating couple: An evaluation of an educational mental health service. *Journal of Counseling Psychology*, *21*(5), 385-389.

Ely, A. L., Guerney, B., Jr., & Stover, L. (1973). Efficacy of the training phase of conjugal therapy. *Psychotherapy: Theory, Research, and Practice*, *10*(3), 201-207.

Figley, C., & Guerney, B., Jr. (1976). *The conjugal relationship enhancement program* (34 minutes, 16mm film; 3/4- or 1/2-inch video). University Park,

The Individual and Family Consultation Center of The Pennsylvania State University.

Giblin, P., Sprenkle, D. H., & Sheehan, R. (1985). Enrichment outcome research: A meta-analysis of premarital, marital and family interventions. *Journal of Marital and Family Therapy, 11*(3), 257-271.

Ginsberg, B. G. (1977). Parent-adolescent relationship development program. In B. G. Guerney, Jr. (Ed.), *Relationship enhancement*. San Francisco: Jossey-Bass.

Ginsberg, B. G., & Vogelsong, E. (1977). Premarital relationship improvement by maximizing empathy and self-disclosure: The PRIMES program. In B. G. Guerney, Jr. (Ed.). *Relationship enhancement*. San Francisco: Jossey-Bass.

Guerney, B., Jr. (Ed.). (1969). *Psychotherapeutic agents: New roles for nonprofessionals, parents and teachers*. New York: Holt, Rinehart, & Winston.

Guerney, B., Jr. (1977a). *Relationship enhancement: Skill training programs for therapy, problem prevention and enrichment*. San Francisco: Jossey-Bass.

Guerney, B., Jr. (1977b). Should teachers treat illiteracy, hypocalligraphy and dysmathematica? *Canadian Counsellor, 12*(1), 9-14.

Guerney, B., Jr. (1982). The delivery of mental health services: Spiritual versus medical versus educational models. In T. R. Vallance & R. M. Sabre (Eds.), *Mental health services in transition: A policy sourcebook*. New York: Human Sciences Press.

Guerney, G., Jr. (1984). Relationship enhancement therapy and training. In D. Larson (Ed.), *Teaching psychological skills: Models for giving psychology away*. Monterey: Brooks/Cole.

Guerney, B., Jr. (1985). *Relationship enhancement: Marital/Family therapist's manual*. State College, PA: IDEALS, P.O. Box 391.

Guerney, B., Jr. (in press). *Relationship enhancement: Clients' manual*. State College, PA: IDEALS, P.O. Box 391.

Guerney, B., Jr., Coufal, J., & Vogelsong, E. (1981). Relationship enhancement versus a traditional approach to therapeutic/preventative/enrichment parent-adolescent programs. *Journal of Consulting and Clinical Psychology, 49*, 927-939.

Guerney, B., Jr., Guerney, L., & Stollak, G. (1971/72). The potential advantages of changing from a medical to an educational model in practicing psychology. *Interpersonal Development, 2*, 238-245.

Guerney, B., Jr., Guerney, L., & Stover, L. (1972). Facilitative therapist attitudes in training parents as psychotherapeutic agents. *The Family Coordinator, 21*(3), 275-278.

Guerney, B., Jr., Stollak, G., & Guerney, L. (1970). A format for a new mode of psychological practice: Or, how to escape a zombie. *The Counseling Psychologist, 2*(2), 97-104.

Guerney, B., Jr., Stollak, G., & Guerney, L. (1971). The practicing psychologist as education – An alternative to the medical practitioner model. *Professional Psychology, 2*(3), 276-282.

Guerney, B., Jr., & Vogelsong, E. (1981). *Relationship enhancement demonstra-*

tion dialogs (audiotapes). University Park: The Individual and Family Consultation Center of The Pennsylvania State University.

Guerney, B., Jr., Vogelsong, E., & Coufal, J. (1983). Relationship enhancement versus a traditional treatment: Follow-up and booster effects. In D. Olson & B. Miller (Eds.), *Family studies review yearbook* (Vol. 1). Beverly Hills: Sage Publications.

Guerney, B., Jr., Vogelsong, E., & Glynn, S. (1977). *Evaluation of the family counseling unit of the Cambria County Probation Bureau*. State College, PA: IDEALS, P.O. Box 391.

Guerney, B., Jr., Vogelsong, E., & Wolfgang, G. (1977). *Foster parent skills training program: First year evaluation*. State College, PA: IDEALS, P.O. Box 391.

Guerney, B., Jr., Wolfgang, G., & Vogelsong, E. (1978). *Foster care systems training project: Second year evaluation*. State College, PA: IDEALS, P.O. Box 391.

Guerney, L. F. (1973). What do you say now? (film). University Park, PA: The Pennsylvania State University in cooperation with the Pennsylvania Department of Public Welfare.

Guerney, L. F. (1974). The training of foster parent trainers (film). University Park, PA: The Pennsylvania State University in cooperation with the Pennsylvania Department of Public Welfare.

Guerney, L. F. (1975). *Foster parent training: A manual for parents*. State College, PA: IDEALS, P.O. Box 391.

Guerney, L. F. (1976a). *Foster parent training: A manual for trainers*. State College, PA: IDEALS, P.O. Box 391.

Guerney, L. F. (1976b). A program for training agency personnel as foster parent trainers. *Child Welfare*, *55*(9), 652-660.

Guerney, L. F. (1977). A description and evaluation of a skills training program for foster parents. *American Journal of Community Psychology*, *5*, 361-371.

Guerney, L. F. (1978). *Parenting: A skills training manual*. State College, PA: IDEALS, P.O. Box 391.

Guerney, L. F. (1983). Introduction to filial therapy. In P. Keller & L. Ritt (Eds.), *Innovations in clinical practice: A source book* (Vol. 2). Sarasota, FL: Professional Resource Exchange.

Guerney, L. F. (in press). *Parent training: A manual for trainers*. State College, PA: IDEALS, P.O. Box 391.

Guerney, L. F., & Wolfgang, G. (1981). Long-range evaluation of effects on foster parents of a foster parent skill training program. *Journal of Clinical Child Psychology*, *10*, 33-37.

Jessee, R., & Guerney, B., Jr. (1981). A comparison of Gestalt and relationship enhancement treatments with married couples. *American Journal of Family Therapy*, *9*, 31-41.

Larson, D. (Ed.). (1984). *Teaching psychological skills: Models for giving psychology away*. Monterey: Brooks/Cole.

Marshall, E. K., & Kurtz, P. D. (Eds.). (1982). *Interpersonal helping skills*. San Francisco: Jossey-Bass.

Matter, M., McAllister, W., & Guerney, B., Jr. [unlisted] (1984). Relationship enhancement for the recovering couple: Working with the intangible. *Focus on Family and Chemical Dependency*, *7*(5), 21-23.

Most, R., & Guerney, B., Jr. (1983). An empirical evaluation of the training of lay volunteer leaders for premarital relationship enhancement. *Family Relations*, *32*, 239-251.

Rappaport, A. F. (1976). Conjugal relationship enhancement program. In D. H. L. Olson (Ed.), *Treating relationships*. Lake Mills, IA: Gtaphic Publishing.

Ross, E., Baker, S., & Guerney, B., Jr. (1984). Effectiveness of relationship enhancement therapy versus therapist's preferred therapy. *American Journal of Family Therapy*, *13*(1), 11-21.

Sensue, M. E. (1981). *Filial therapy follow-up study: Effects on parental acceptance and child adjustment*. Unpublished doctoral dissertation, The Pennsylvania State University.

Sywulak, A. E. (1977). *The effect of filial therapy on parental acceptance and child adjustment*. Unpublished doctoral dissertation, The Pennsylvania State University.

Sywulak, A. E. (1984). Creating a whole atmosphere in a group home for retarded adolescents. *Academic Psychology Bulletin*, *6*, 325-327.

Vogelsong, E., & Guerney, G., Jr. (1978). The relationship enhancement program for family therapy and enrichment (45 minutes, 16mm film; 3/4- or 1/2-inch video). University Park, PA: The Individual and Family Consultation Center of The Pennsylvania State University.

Vogelsong, E., & Guerney, B., Jr. (1979). Filial therapy (40 minutes, 16mm film; 3/4- or 1/2-inch video). University Park, PA: The Individual and Family Consultation Center of The Pennsylvania State University.

Vogelsong, E., & Guerney, B., Jr. (1980). Working with parents of disturbed adolescents. In R. R. Abidin (Ed.), *Parent education and intervention handbook*. Springfield, IL: Charles C Thomas, Publisher.

Vogelsong, E., Guerney, B., Jr., & Guerney, L. F. (1983). Relationship enhancement therapy with inpatients and their families. In R. Luber & C. Anderson (Eds.), *Communication training approaches to family intervention with psychiatric patients*. New York: Human Sciences Press.

Wieman, R. J. (1973). *Conjugal relationship modification and reciprocal reinforcement: A comparison of treatments for marital discord*. Unpublished doctoral dissertation, The Pennsylvania State University.

Home Visits: An Effective Strategy for Engaging the Involuntary Client

Pallassana R. Balgopal
Michael A. Patchner
Charles H. Henderson

ABSTRACT. This paper presents an in-depth analysis of home visits as an effective strategy for engaging involuntary clients into treatment and making treatment more effective. More specifically, this study examines the effects that regularly planned home visits have upon engagement in and attitudes toward parenting training of protective service clients. The home visits not only produced high attendance rates and low dropout rates but caused the participants to be more favorably disposed toward learning the knowledge and skills taught in the parenting program. Because of the home visits, participants were more engaged in the treatment program and were, consequently, better able to benefit.

Frequently clients who receive child welfare services have virtually no say as to the relevancy or the mode of services offered. It is infrequent that this involuntary status is recognized. Usually they tend to be labeled as resistive and hostile clients. The crucial variable affecting the individual's induction into the role of client is the manner through which he/she is perceived by the worker and the agency.

During the formative phase of social work profession, home visits was an integral part of the professional activity. The "Friendly

---

Pallassana R. Balgopal, Michael A. Patchner, and Charles H. Henderson are affiliated with the School of Social Work, University of Illinois, Urbana, IL 61801.

Visitor" went to the clients' home to assess their living situation and home environment. Such visits continue to be regarded as an important assessment tool for gathering new and pertinent data through observation of the client's milieu and their interactional patterns.

The focus of this paper is to present an in-depth analysis of home visits as an effective strategy for engaging involuntary clients into treatment. More specifically, it examines the effect that regularly planned home visits have upon engagement in and attitudes toward parenting training of protective service clients of child welfare agencies.

INVOLUNTARY CLIENTS

The social work profession, despite its commitment to the general welfare of all citizens, and its adherence to such values as human worth and dignity, self-determination, nonjudgmental attitude, and democratic principles, has not succeeded in convincing the society at large that a large number of individuals who seek their services are often in their plight due to reasons beyond their control. They are frequently victims of social, economic and political oppression which is further extenuated by institutional racism and sexism. Clients are frequently seen as unnecessarily dependent on publicly and privately supported social services. Social work profession is also blamed for nurturing the clients' dependency. In a society where the Protestant Work Ethic is still considered an essential virtue, those who are unable to pull themselves up by their bootstraps are looked down upon, and considerable stigma is attached for their dependency. Social work clients often find themselves in a no-win situation.

Although the voluntary-involuntary status of clients is relative, the contention is that all social work clients are basically involuntary. The authors believe that people have the potential to decide their own destiny, and that basically they are good, independent, and industrious. Thus a majority of clients including those who seek social services voluntarily do so with a degree of discomfort, shame, and guilt. The voluntary-involuntary status of clients is determined by the process through which they were inducted in the role of a client. Attention to the involuntary status of clients and how they affect social work practice has been minimal, although there are exceptions (Etzioni, 1961; Briar & Miller, 1971; Yelaja, 1971; Hepworth & Larsen, 1982; Balgopal & Vassil, 1983; Cingolari, 1984). The involuntary induction of individuals into client roles is often associated with authoritarian settings such as child welfare, public welfare, and correctional agencies. Etzioni (1961), as discussed by Balgopal and Vassil (1983), has succinctly identified three categories through which processes of involuntary induction are instituted:

1. *Alienative Involvement*: In this category, clients seldom share the worker's values and often are hostile to compliance with agency and worker expectations. Examples of these include protective service clients of child welfare agencies, inmates in correctional institutions, members in substance abuse programs, and children in remedial centers of learning.
2. *Calculative Involvement*: This category encompasses a quid pro quo orientation that is nested within a win-lose situation. The clients knowingly permit themselves to be "taken in as clients," and in the same process maintain control over the situation. For example, spouses of alcoholics will often "play the game" of presenting as clients, whereas in reality they are hesitant to give up their control over their partners.
3. *Moral Involvement*: When client and worker expectations are complementary, the involvement of the client is manifested in a high degree of cooperation and commitment to mutually shared expectations. Both workers and clients are clear of what each has to offer and to work on. Married couples who seek and accept the terms of assistance in the resolution of their marital difficulties illustrate this point.

HOME VISITS

As indicated earlier, visits to a client's home were an integral part of social workers' professional activity. As much as it was well intended, these home visits came under criticism as workers' encroachment on the client's privacy. Some of this criticism was justified especially when public welfare workers visited their clients' homes with punitive intentions to check out whether the clients were honest and not cheating the welfare departments. This policing function of social workers is resented by the clients, and understandably so.

As social work gained societal acceptance as a profession, most social workers became concerned with preserving their hard earned status. They resisted being categorized as the "friendly visitor" and the "do gooder." In their struggle to preserve the professional status one of the significant moves was to eliminate the practice of visiting their clients in their own homes. In the last two decades professionally trained social workers have been increasingly office-based practitioners. Visiting clients in their homes is virtually limited to child welfare, public welfare, and corrections whose personnel are seldom professionally trained. Unfortunately by eliminating the practice of home visits from their repertoire of strategies of interventions, social work is giving up a powerful and effective tool of working with their clients. Home visits have unlimited potential for working effectively with diversified social work clientele.

Cohen and Egan (1981) in discussing social work home visits in health settings indicate that such visits provide information through observation of the home environment and yields previously unavailable information. Clients are less likely to be defensive in their own homes, and derive comfort from familiar surroundings, feelings of control, self-image re-enhancement and a sense of relief that a social worker has come to their home to help.

Axelrod (1978) suggests that with the recognition of home care as an effective means of preventing or postponing costly institutionalizations, health care agencies will require the services of professionally trained social workers more than ever. Two major legislations have significantly influenced this trend toward community care. The Community Mental Health Act of 1963 mandated that each community must provide certain mental health services, including crisis outreach services to persons in their homes. The Medicare amendments to Social Security Act of 1965 included allowances for reimbursement of social work services, when provided by professionally trained staff within a certified home health agency.

Moynihan (1974) in assessing the relevancy of home visits for family treatment delineates six areas of benefit from visits by professional social workers to clients' homes, and they are: (1) The caseworker becomes the family caseworker. Family members are not singled out as the focus of treatment. (2) Children's fantasies about treatment are exposed and clarified. (3) Strengths of the family are emphasized and visual observation is made of family atmosphere, values and investment. (4) Home visitation early in the contact with the client is an immediate and concrete offer to help, which implies a willingness and interest of the worker to extend himself/herself. (5) Home visitation reinforces the worker's willingness to risk himself/herself on the family's terms. (6) Home visitation facilitates increased cooperation from all the members of the client family.

Schlachter (1975) proposes that in working with adolescents and their parents, home visits are a preferable approach to seeing the clients in the office. He points out that by seeing the parties in their own home, the practitioner can assess the "turf" of both the adolescents and their parents. Adolescents are much more comfortable when seen in their homes. Parents do not have to worry about getting the adolescents to the appointment, and when seen at home, fathers are frequently present and can be included in the discussion. By visiting clients' homes the social worker can assess the neighborhood and available community resources.

In a recent article Holbrook (1983) proposes that social workers through their home visits can provide social evidence of the impact of the massive cuts in social programs on the lives of the poor. He suggests that such objective reporting can once again be utilized to educate the community and to mobilize the public toward social reform, and put an end to the arbitrary discontinuation of essential services to the needy.

The benefits of home visits as discussed in the literature are apparent. They are seen as the primary tool for gathering information and making a comprehensive assessment. There is minimal evidence showing the systematic analysis of this strategy for improving involuntary clients' attitudes toward interventions and actively engaging them in the treatment process. This study is designed to assess the impact of home visits on these two dimensions.

METHODOLOGY

Data were gathered from 34 abusive and neglective parents who participated in a parent training program which was held in three different locations in Central Illinois. All but three of these participants had a history of unwillingness to acknowledge their problems as abusive parents. They were reluctant recipients of services geared toward altering their dysfunctional behaviors. Given this reluctance to accept themselves as abusive and their lack of motivation to engage in the helping process, these participants clearly fit into Etzioni's category of "Alienative Involvement."

The training program, focusing upon parenting skills, consisted of a two-hour session held once a week for eight weeks, and regularly scheduled home visits. The curriculum for the training sessions included lectures, discussions, and homework, and centered on effective strategies for communicating, building self-esteem, controlling angry feelings, and managing children's behavior.

A contract was established which included the following: participants agreed to work on self-identified goals to enhance their parenting skills; participants would attend at least six out of the eight training sessions; they were to notify the trainer in advance when they would not be able to attend a session; they would be present for the scheduled times of the home visits; and the information gathered during the home visits and training sessions would not be shared with the referring agency's work or become part of their official record.

A home visit was made prior to the beginning of the sessions and four other times at two-week intervals during the eight-week training period. The home visits were designed to provide individual attention to program participants and their families in order for them to discuss their particular situation and problems, to enhance their learning of the material presented in the training sessions, and to build upon needed parenting skills as identified in the initial contract. The home visits also provided pertinent information about the participants' environment and allowed for the training to become more relevant.

The training program was specifically structured for state child welfare clients who were abusive or neglective parents. These clients were recommended as needing assistance in developing parenting skills. Of the parents in this study, 91% were state child welfare clients and nine percent were referred from other sources such as mental health centers, schools, or self-referrals.

At the beginning of the initial training session the participants were given a pre-test consisting of two identical semantic differential scales which measured participants' attitudes about having home visits and participating in the parent training. The semantic differential scales included 16 bipolar adjectives rated along a seven-point continuum. The maximum value of seven was given for the most positive response and a value of one for the most negative. When an item within the scale was not responded to a middle value of four was assigned. Responses for the 16 items were added together to create a total scale score with a possible range from 16 to 112. The post-test instrument also included a number of items to ascertain demographic information and several open-ended questions related to expectations and concerns about both the home visits and the training. At the conclusion of the training participants were administered the same instrument and were asked to evaluate the home visits and the training sessions.

Sample

Of the three training groups, one had 14 participants and the others had ten each. The demographic characteristics of the participants varied regarding their sex, age, education, income, and the number of adults and children in the family. The participants were mostly female (68%) and ranged in age from 18 to 56 with a median age of 31. Their educational background was mixed with 48% graduating from high school or completing the G.E.D., 17% having some college and the remaining 35% dropping out from school anywhere from the eighth through the eleventh grades. Two-thirds of the participants had two adults living in their home, while 17% had only one and 17% more than two. The number of children in each home ranged from one to five with each participant having on the average of 2.6 children living with them. The ages of the children were evenly distributed and ranged from a few months to over 19 years. Only 18% of the participants had annual family incomes of

$25,000 or more, while 65% had incomes less than $10,000 per year.

FINDINGS

Engagement in Treatment

The caseworkers who made the referrals to the training program indicated that their clients resented the role of the child welfare agencies in their lives and would be resistant to participate in any treatment program. The caseworkers cautioned that such resistance and resentment would be present during the training program. Such feelings were indeed evidenced during the first home visit. However, after clarifying the purpose of the training and establishing the contract the participants became less guarded. The home visits actually helped create favorable attitudes toward the training and helped cause the participants to have more realistic expectations of what could be accomplished by the training program. These positive attitudes and expectations were demonstrated by the scores on the pretest instrument. Subsequent home visits further contributed toward their feelings about the parent training program.

The home visits further enhanced the motivation of the participants to attend the training sessions. The participants contracted to attend at least six out of the eight training sessions which would give an attendance rate of 75%. The overall attendance rate was 83%—much above what was expected. When the participants did miss a session, they notified the trainers in advance and gave legitimate reasons for not attending, such as their children being ill, a change in their work schedule, or personal commitments which were made before the training had been scheduled. Moreover, the dropout rate for these individuals was only six percent which is extremely low given this type of client population (Balgopal and Vassil, 1983). Those that did withdraw from the training program did so because of moving from the area or having a setback in their health.

The home visits not only produced high attendance rates and low dropout rates but caused the participants to be more favorably disposed toward learning the knowledge and skills taught in the parenting program. Because of the home visits the participants were more engaged in the treatment program and were consequently better able to benefit.

Attitudes About Home Visits and Training Sessions

Most of the participants came to the initial training session with positive expectations and attitudes regarding the parent training program. Initially they were slightly more favorable about the training sessions and less so about the home visits. Overall they scored an average of 76.9 on the semantic differential scale which measured their attitudes toward having home visits and 80.5 on the semantic differential scale which measured their attitudes about the training sessions. On both of these scales the pre-test totals ranged from the lowest possible score of 16 to the highest possible score of 112.

Their major expectations about the training sessions were that they would learn better ways of communicating with their children, controlling their temper, disciplining their children, handling particular behavior problems, and generally being a better parent. They expected that the home visits would be a vehicle by which they would receive individual attention and help with making the skills learned in training sessions work in their homes. The participants felt that the home visits would provide a realistic perspective of the problems and would give them an opportunity to discuss on a one-to-one basis in the relaxed atmosphere of their home. One client generally reflected the participants' expectations by reporting that the home visits would provide "a full cycle of communication."

The participants were not without reservations about the training program and home visits. They reported that they had concerns whether the knowledge gained in the sessions could realistically be applied to their personal situations and some even questioned whether the information presented would be effective at all. They had even more deep-rooted concerns about the home visits. Some felt uncomfortable about someone coming to their "dirty, messy house" while others were concerned about how spouses and other family members would react to a stranger coming into their home talking about family problems. The primary concern about the home visits was that participants did not want anyone coming into their homes to "check on" them. Many felt that home visits would be an intrusion of their privacy.

The data collected at the end of the training program showed that none of their concerns materialized. The participants felt that they did learn practical ways of parenting from the training and they were helped with their problems. Many felt that by attending the sessions they were better able to communicate with and understand their children. Moreover, participants felt relieved to realize they were not alone in having problems with their children.

The home visits proved to be extremely beneficial to the participants because they felt that someone was truly interested in them and the problems they were having. They were not only able to discuss the material presented in training sessions, but they were able to integrate it into their daily lives. They believed that the personal goals that they had established for themselves were realized through the home visits. Some participants even expressed that they wanted more and would have liked to have continued the home visits even after the program had ended. The participants also indicated that because of the support and positive reinforcement they received during the home visits they were able to be freer in sharing their concerns about parenting deficits. In other words these visits were instrumental in facilitating participation in the group sessions.

The scores on the post-test regarding the training sessions averaged 95.8 and ranged from 64 to 112 while the scores on the post-test about the home visits averaged 92.6 with an identical range from 64 to 112. The increases in the scores from the pre-test to the post-test were statistically significant (see Table 1). The semantic differential scale score which measured attitudes about the training

TABLE 1

ATTITUDES TOWARD PARENT TRAINING SESSIONS AND HOME VISITS

Semantic Differential Scale	Pre-test $\bar{x}$	Post-test $\bar{x}$	T Value	DF	Probability
Attitudes Toward Home Visits	76.9	92.6	-3.38	33	.002
Attitudes Toward Parent Training Sessions	80.6	95.8	-3.31	33	.002

sessions increased from an average of 80.6 on the pre-test to 95.8 on the post-test and the semantic differential scale score measuring attitudes about the training increased from a mean of 76.9 to 92.6.

Overall, the pre-test showed that the participants in the parent training program were favorably disposed to it, but had some major reservations about the home visits and the usefulness of the training sessions. After attending the sessions and having the home visits their attitudes became even more positive and they realized that their concerns never materialized.

DISCUSSION AND IMPLICATIONS

The findings of this study clearly reflect that home visits were instrumental in creating a positive disposition and an active engagement of these clients into treatment. These clients generally had perceived visits to their homes by professionals as interfering in their personal lives and lifestyle. This change in the clients' attitudes can be attributed to reasons such as: home visits were scheduled to assist clients to work on their individual goals, and the purpose of these visits were complementary to the overall goals of the parenting training. The social control aspects of such home visits by child welfare workers for these clients, which often include monitoring parenting roles, were not the intent of these visits. Due to the absence of this function the participants immediately became less defensive and on their own volition shared their concerns and deficiencies of their parenting roles and sought guidance in this regard. Such sharing of concerns and voluntarily seeking assistance was also evidenced in the training sessions which soon evolved as a mutual help and support group.

Due to the small portion of participants (9%) in this study who were regarded as "voluntary," no specific comparisons were made between the two types of participants. Nonetheless, the findings supported the assumption that systematically planned and structured home visits can be a significant factor for engaging involuntary clients into treatment. To further examine these findings more study is needed to compare voluntary and involuntary clients and to test the lasting impact that home visits make upon their attitudes to treatment and their relationship with the agency's workers.

REFERENCES

Axelrod, T. B. (1978). Innovative roles for social workers in home care programs. *Health and Social Work*, *3*(3), 48-66.

Balgopal, P. R., & Vassil, T. V. (1983). *Groups in social work: An ecological perspective*. New York: MacMillan Publishing Company.

Briar, S., & Miller. H. (1971). *Problems and issues in social casework*. New York: Columbia University Press.

Cingolani, J. (1984). Social conflict perspective on work with involuntary clients. *Social Work*, *29*(5), 442-446.

Cohen, S. N., & Egan, B. (1981). The social work home visit in a health care setting. *Social Work in Health Care*, *6*(4), 55-67.

Etzioni, A. A. (1961). *Comparative analysis of complete organizations*. New York: The Free Press.

Hepworth, D. H., & Larsen, J. A. (1982). *Direct social work practice*. Homewood, IL: Dorsey Press.

Holbrook, T. (1983). Going among them: The evolution of the home visit. *Journal of Sociology and Social Welfare*, *10*(1), 112-135.

Moynihan, S. (1974). Home visits for family treatment. *Social Casework*, *55*(10), 612-617.

Schlachter, R. H. (1975). Home counseling of adolescents and parents. *Social Work*, *20*(6), 427-428, 481.

Yelaja, S. A. (1971). *Authority and social work: Concept and the use*. Toronto: University of Toronto Press.

The Entrance of Systems Family Therapy into a Residential Treatment Center

William J. Matthews
Janine Roberts

ABSTRACT. The following paper outlines the impact of introducing a different theoretical orientation to behavioral change (systemic/strategic family therapy) at an adolescent residential treatment center which had been primarily psychodynamic in orientation. The introduction of a strategic and systemic approach in this setting is discussed in terms of an initial description of the agency homeostasis followed by a description of the family therapy models employed. The final section of the paper presents suggestions for introducing youth care workers to systems thinking in conjunction with a specific approach to training youth care staff in the techniques of systemic strategic work.

Imber-Coppersmith (1983) indicated that as families show redundant behavioral patterns that maintain an equilibrium so, too, do larger systems such as mental health agencies show similar tendencies toward homeostasis. Held (1982) suggested that the professional entering the mental health system is analogous to the family therapist entering the family system. This entry is often difficult and resistance to change is frequently experienced by the therapist. Both Imber-Coppersmith (1983) and Held (1982) suggested that the systems oriented family therapist must consider the family and the context (line staff, supervisors, agency) in which the therapy is to occur in order for therapy to succeed. Held (1982) indicated that the inter-

---

William J. Matthews and Janine Roberts are affiliated with the Counseling Psychology Program, School of Education, University of Massachusetts, Amherst, MA 01003. The authors would like to thank Evan Imber-Coppersmith for her helpful comments on this manuscript.

ventions used in family systems work (e.g., avoidance of triangulation, going slowly, taking a one-down complementary position, reframing, etc.) are not only applicable to the larger system but, in fact, may be quite necessary to insure the success of therapy and the effectiveness of the therapist within the system.

The present article has two purposes: (1) to describe the homeostatic patterns in a residential treatment center for adolescents and (2) to present a training strategy in the systems approach to change for youth care staff which is designed to gain acceptance for family work.

THE AGENCY

The Valley Children's Center (VCA, a pseudonym) was created for the treatment needs of adolescents in 1976. The agency consists of senior management (executive director, director of clinical services, and program director) clinical staff, school staff and residential house staff. There are separate residences for the adolescent girls and boys. Each residence contains approximately 6-8 clients, 4 youth care workers per shift and a head of residence. In addition each residence has one clinician assigned to it. The program also includes a psychoeducationally oriented school (approximately 8 teachers) in which school attendance is mandatory. The total client population is relatively small and serves approximately 25-28 adolescents at any one time. Clients in the program typically manifest difficulties in: family relationships; peer relationships; school achievement, and self-esteem.

In the early development of the program role boundaries between clinicians, teachers, and youth care workers were not always clear. Teachers and youth care workers, often out of necessity, were involved in a great deal of counseling and behavioral management. Clinicians were frequently called in to assist teachers during school crises. Much of the therapeutic work was accomplished more as a function of the staff member's personal charisma with a client than as a function of a formal theoretical treatment model. Client management was often based on the value placed on the personal relationships with a staff by the client.

ENTRANCE OF FAMILY THERAPY TO THE AGENCY

The initial family work consisted primarily of the clinician making contact with the family around visitation, program rules, allowances, clothing and case management. On some occasions the clinician would visit the family in the home if the family would not or could not come to the agency. In much of the early work, the clinician tended to focus on the "rules of how good families live." The therapeutic modality at the agency was primarily individual in orientation.

As the agency became more established in the mental health community, the clinical focus of the program changed towards a more formal structure and theoretical base. The epistemological *zeitgeist* of the agency developed toward a linear cause-effect model in which insight was considered to be a major precursor to change. The consulting psychiatrist was traditionally trained and psychoanalytically oriented.

The director of clinical services having recognized the need for more formal family work and the lack of trained family therapists hired a family therapy consultant. The family therapy consultant operated from a systems epistemology and utilized the work of the Mental Research Institute (Watzlawick et al., 1974), the Milan Group (Selvini-Palazzoli et al., 1978) and a structural approach to families (Minuchin, 1974). The introduction of a consultant with a different theoretical orientation towards therapeutic change was initially disruptive to the homeostasis of the agency.

Imber-Coppersmith (1983) postulated three basic rules that support the larger system's homeostatic patterns. These "rules" have utility in considering the effect of introducing a different model of change to the VCA.

Conflictual Triads Within the Agency

Because there was a great deal of involvement by the various components within the agency there were often conflicts between these components. The conflicts frequently centered around responsibility for the client and who should have decision-making power. For example, a client may violate a house rule before school and be kept in the house to make a correction in the problem. This response by the house would be disruptive to the school procedure and often resulted in friction between the units. There were a number of dysfunctional triads that occurred within the agency. One type of dysfunctional triad involved the client, the family and the agency. Often there would be an alliance between the agency and client against the family or the client and family would align against the agency. Another dysfunctional triadic relationship which developed with the entrance of family therapy to the agency involved the house staff, client and the family therapist. The house staff were initially resistant to family work often because of the blame directed toward the family for the client problems and/or the fear that family therapy would be upsetting to the client and be disruptive to the residence. Thus, the house staff and client would often align against the family therapist. Such alignment would be in the form of undercutting the family work, challenging of the family therapist's work, avoidance of sessions by the client.

Everyone Has a Piece of the Client

Another problem encountered by the systems oriented family therapist at the VCA was the wide-ranging involvement with the client by each of the components within the agency (e.g., head of residence, youth care workers, teachers and individual clinicians). In addition, there were often community agencies involved with the client's family (e.g., welfare, school, probation officer). Such involvement was often stressful for the client and/or family and served to diffuse boundaries between client/family and the larger system. This diffusion helps maintain the larger system in a complementary one-up position in relationship to the client/family (Imber-Coppersmith, 1983).

Someone Needs to Be Blamed

Staff at the VCA tended to blame the adolescent and/or the adolescent's family for the adolescent's problems. The nonblaming stance and the notion of mutually influencing causality in systems therapy challenged the concept of linear blame held by the staff. Most of the staff believed that the purpose of therapy was to "fix" the client. Thus, the staff considered family therapy to be another treatment modality whose purpose was to fix the client's family. Imber-Coppersmith (1983) stated that such a shift from individual blame to family blame is, in fact, no shift at all. A blaming stance may allow the blamer to be in a one-up position relative to the blamed, however, such a stance ignores mutually influencing interaction and is unlikely to lead to second order change.

An attempt at resolution of the above "rules" is presented in the final section of this article which discusses youth care worker training in systems thinking.

THREE MODELS OF FAMILY TREATMENT EMPLOYED

Three approaches to family treatment were employed by the authors at the VCA: (1) Brief Therapy (Watzlawick, Weakland, & Fisch, 1974; Weakland, Fisch, & Watzlawick, 1974; and Fisch, Weakland, & Segal, 1983); (2) Long Brief Therapy (Selvini-Palazzoli, 1974, 1978; Selvini-Palazzoli, Cecchin, Parata, & Boscolo, 1978); and (3) Structural Family Therapy (Minuchin, Rosman, & Baker, 1978).

While these approaches to family work have differences, Roberts (1979) has indicated that there are some important commonalities: (1) A systems view of family interaction. Behavior is governed by interpersonal interactions. Thus, the emphasis is on family rules that govern the patterns of interaction. There is a shift from an intrapsychic view of causation to looking at what function the symptom or problem plays in the whole family. (2) Change occurs as a function of shifts in interactional patterns as opposed to insight. (3) Behavior is seen as ahistorical. The importance of past traumas or "causes" are de-emphasized and a model of circular causality is adopted. (4) Homework is given between family sessions as a way of promoting pattern shifts and extending the influence of therapy. (5) The family therapist utilizes the language of the family and meets the family at their model of the world. A brief overview of each approach will be presented.

Brief Therapy Model

This approach to family therapy is symptom focused with the goal of the therapy to bring symptom relief. Small changes are seen as enough to initiate larger changes in the family system, therefore, the therapy focuses on small pragmatic alterations that bring indirect change to the family organization.

Problems are seen as difficulties that have arisen in normal day-to-day interactions, in particular, in transitional steps in the family such as a child entering school or the first child moving out of the home, etc. Families sometime become stuck in a rigid negative feedback pattern when they do not move onto the next developmental stage. Thus, this approach utilizes interventions that are designed to interrupt the feedback cycles that have become established. Interventions are typically indirect and are developed in relationship to what the family offers. Their symptom and world view are accepted first, then the therapist works toward small changes. This model contends that small changes open up new possibilities in resolving the day-to-day transitional patterns of family life. The interventions of the Brief Therapy Model (e.g., paradoxical instructions, reframing, illusion of alternatives) will be explained in relationship to training youth care staff in their use.

Long Brief Therapy

The word "brief" refers to a time limited contract between the therapist and the family similar to the Brief Model previously discussed and "long" refers to the length of time in between family sessions (approximately a month).

The Milan group does not just focus on symptom eradication but focuses on changing family rules since in their view, the symptom is seen as functional in the organization of the family system. The Milan group feels that if they are successful in changing one fundamental rule in the family, then change will take place in the family interaction patterns. The interaction of the family is described as a game and the therapist's interventions provide a counter game with different rules. In the Milan view, power in the family game does not belong to any one individual member, rather the power is in the rules of the game. In a dysfunctional family, changing the rules from within the family is difficult. Often change can be facilitated by someone outside the system who can meta-communicate on changing the rules.

Milan approach has a distinctive style to the individual session which is: (1) the presession—a discussion among team members; (2) the interview—the therapist interviews the family while the therapeutic team observes from behind a one-way mirror; (3) the intersession—discussion among team members while the family waits; (4) the intervention—the conclusions of the team are delivered to the family while the team observes; and (5) the postsession—a discussion amongst team members (Tomm, 1981). The Milan group employs such powerful interventions as positive connotation, symptom prescriptions, rituals and therapist impotence. (The interventions of positive connotation and symptom prescription will be discussed in relationship to the training of the youth care staff.) An importance difference between the MRI and the Milan group is that the Milan group does not just focus on a behavior or set of behaviors, their interventions are designed to include the social matrix of relationships in which the behaviors occur.

Structural Family Therapy

Unlike the MRI group who start at the most specific level and work out, Minuchin starts at the abstract level and works in (Hoffman, 1981). The structural approach as discussed by Minuchin (1974) postulates a normative model for a well functioning family. Thus, a well functioning family has clearly marked boundaries. The marital subsystem has closed boundaries to protect the privacy of the spouses. The parental subsystem has clear boundaries that allow the access necessary for effective parenting. The sibling subsystem is hierarchically organized according to sex and age as determined by the family's culture.

With this model in mind, the therapist has the task of noting the deviance between it and the family in therapy (Hoffman, 1981). From this theoretical orientation, therapy consists of restructuring the family organization so that it will approximate this normative model more closely (Hoffman, 1981). Subsequent to successful joining with the family, restructuring techniques can bring about change. Minuchin delineates seven categories of restructuring: marking boundaries, actualizing family transactional patterns, escalating stress, utilizing symptoms, assigning tasks, manipulating mood, and supporting, educating or guiding (Minuchin, 1974).

A structural family assessment is done after the first session in order to examine the family subsystems, boundaries hierarchy and capacity for restructuring. In addition to the use of a structural family map, a genogram detailing the family's three generational relationship system is also obtained (Guerin & Pendagast, 1976). These two assessment techniques help the therapist form a picture of the family's characteristics. The use of structural maps and genograms will also be discussed in relationship to youth care staff training.

TRAINING YOUTH CARE STAFF IN THE SYSTEMIC FAMILY THERAPY MODEL

As was previously discussed, the effectiveness of therapy is related to its environmental context. An important part of that context was the youth care staff. Their reluctance towards family therapy was understandable. Anything that increased the difficulty of an already difficult job could be expected to be met with little enthusiasm. The authors believed that in order for family therapy to be effective, not only was the support of the youth care staff necessary, but providing training to youth care workers would only increase their professional effectiveness and thereby enhance the effectiveness of the agency.

The following is a description of the training that one unit of the VCA received, and how they then applied that training to their day-to-day work with the adolescents in residence at the agency. The unit consists of a staff of nine youth care workers. They work in two groups, with each group working four days of the week, 40 hours a week, at Clare House (a pseudonym), the residence for seven young women.

Each residential house has a therapist connected to it who sees each of the clients living there for individual therapy on a weekly basis. This therapist/case manager also coordinates the treatment for their families. The therapist may, in fact, provide direct clinical service to the family or perhaps be behind the one-way mirror as part of the team working with that family. This clinician is also defined as a consultant to the unit who, working in conjunction with the Househead, is available to help examine group interactions, answer staff questions, and provide direction for the milieu treatment of a particular resident.

Training began when the clinician secured permission from the Househead and Program Staff to have a 45-minute block of time most weeks during the regular staff meeting when all the Clare staff except for the night staff met. This time was requested so that there would be a regular, planful way to introduce new ideas into the house. The support of the Househead for the use of this time was invaluable. The following training was done during this time.

First, the therapist began by showing excerpts of videos from family sessions of young women in the house. (All families are asked to sign a release which gives the agency permission to videotape family sessions and to use the videos for treatment and training purposes within the agency.) The purpose of this was threefold. One objective was to demonstrate to the staff the family context in which the people with whom they were working had their "symptoms." A second purpose was to get support and understanding for the family work—to educate staff about it. A final purpose was to begin to demonstrate some family therapy techniques. For instance, with one resistant family, the therapist frequently used the technique of "illusion of alternatives." The therapist would ask the family if they would like to meet again the following Tuesday or Thursday, not offering them a choice of no meeting at all. Or the therapist might ask the family whether they wanted to address a particular issue at the beginning of the session, or the middle of the session. Excerpts of videos were chosen that demonstrated particular techniques, so that over time the techniques of relabeling and reframing, positive connotation, prescribing of symptoms, confusion technique, shingling, directives in therapy session, use of metaphors, homework directives, rituals and prescriptions were all shown.

As the staff become more comfortable with these types of interventions, they were asked to think of ways that they could apply these techniques in the house. For instance, in the seemingly simple area of house chores, staff realized that they could save themselves a lot of conflict by following the lead of the therapist above. Rather than asking the kids, "When do you want to do your chore?", they began to say things like, "Do you want to do your chore this afternoon or this evening?" "O.K., you want to do it this evening. Do you want to do it at 7:00 or 8:00?"

Then, as the video excerpts of families were shown, the clinician began to introduce the structural maps (Minuchin, 1974) and genograms (Guerin & Pendagast, 1976) of the families that were being viewed. The goal of this effort was to teach staff how to use the genogram and structural map to easily codify information on a family system. Many of these cases on which we worked involved multi-generational families. The genogram has been an important tool to expand the framework of the structural map. As the maps and genograms were of families with whom they often interacted, the staff indicated a high degree of interest. The therapist began to relate specific goals in the therapy to the hierarchy, boundaries, subsystems, generations, stage in life cycle and placement on a continuum of enmeshment/disengagement shown on the structural maps and genograms.

At this point some supplemental readings were made available for people to pass informally in the house, and then discussed in the staff meetings. Included were some chapters from Haley's (1976) *Problem Solving Therapy* and excerpts from a paper by one of the authors of this article which summarized, compared, and contrasted two strategic models and the structural model of Minuchin (Roberts, 1979). As time went on, other readings were circulated including articles by Jesse and L'Abate (1980) and Bergman (1980). Staff members who wanted to do more reading were referred to Watzlawick (1979), Weakland et al. (1974) and Selvini-Palazzoli et al. (1978). A bibliography of readings on family therapy was made available.

Simple and powerful exercises to demonstrate the strength of a system were done with the staff of the unit. These exercises also helped bring the staff together as a group.

One of the first of these exercises was role-playing a family, then adding a symptomatic member to the family and seeing how this affected the family roles, rules, organization, and functioning. Another was an exercise creating a moving machine with a group of three or four people. Each machine was then analyzed in terms of an open system, closed system, feedback loops, homeostasis, boundaries, hierarchy, how people could get in and out of it, and its interface with the outside world. Some nonverbal art exercises were done to demonstrate the power of body language. In one, for example, participants created a picture by blowing food coloring through straws, and they were asked to examine their roles in the exercise in terms of symmetry and complementarity (Watzlawick, Weakland, & Fisch, 1974). Group games from Pfeiffer and Jones (1970) and theatre games from Spolin (1968) were also used to demonstrate systems concepts.

The experiential component along with the video segments illustrated very dramatically some of the concepts behind strategic/systemic family therapy. The exercises were a crucial part of the training, in conjunction with the more didactic information.

Next, the youth care workers were taught how to apply the structural map by drawing structural maps to show the dynamics of Clare House. These maps included themselves, the clients, the therapist, and the Househead. This was a chance to anchor-in the skills of actually creating the map (using the symbols, what information to use in the assessment) as well as a way for them to begin to look at the house as a system and what type of changes may be appropriate for that system. This became a particularly useful tool when new kids entered the house or kids graduated as these were always times of major shifts in interactional patterns in the residence.

As described earlier, youth care staff began creating their own programs in the house. For instance, when scapegoating became covertly prevalent in Clare House and the group evidenced a strong need for one of their peers to be on the bottom of their hierarchy, "Zelda Scapegoat" (a dummy dressed in the clothing of a teenage girl) was created. Attention was directed to Zelda when scapegoating was occurring, to make the covert, overt (Watzlawick et al., 1974). Thus, the scapegoating manuever became more difficult to play.

House staff sophistication with these techniques grew to a very high level. A 19-year-old female—one of the oldest clients in the agency – is an illustrative example of this point. This client would often engage in immature, unfocused, demanding behavior. The staff labeled this behavior as "flaky." The senior shift worker identified this behavior as important and necessary to the girl (positive connotation), and therefore prescribed specific times in which she must act "flaky" (symptom prescription from Watzlawick et al., 1974). When the girl acted "flaky" at times other than the designated times, she was told to stop and reminded of her scheduled times. When the scheduled times occurred, she was reminded of the behavior she needed to show. In a very short time, she refused to act "flaky" at the prescribed time or any other time.

The paradoxical technique of presenting particular behavior was a direct translation of symptom prescription in strategic family work. The staff's use of this technique with this particular client represented both a sophisticated understanding and intervention with a difficult problem.

The openness and willingness of the staff to consider alternative solutions to difficult problems was nicely demonstrated in the case of a verbally abusive and somewhat hysterical 17-year-old female. The family work was oriented toward strengthening the parental subsystem while placing the client in a more age appropriate role within the family. It became obvious to the therapist that placing the parents in charge of the client during the session would often result in the client storming out of therapy back to the residence. When back in the residence, the client would often be disruptive to the unit. The therapist began to inform the house staff of an upcoming family session and indicated that a particular topic of discussion would probably result in the client storming out of therapy back to the residence. House staff in conjunction with the therapist began to predict to the client that this would happen and that such behavior was reflective of her present developmental level which was perhaps much younger than her chronological age. She was further told (in the sessions) that such behavior needed to happen as it provided her parents an opportunity to parent her and the agency an opportunity to care for her as it would a younger child. Such a prediction by the house staff and therapist was not going to be given confirmation by her. She quickly stopped the storming out of the session.

The house staff employed another family therapy technique with the same client who had the habit at the end of therapy sessions or house meetings of making rather dramatic and upsetting announcements or complaints. Rather than attempting to stop this behavior, which did not work, in both the therapy sessions and house meetings this behavior was prescribed for her at the beginning of the sessions or meeting. She was told that she needed to take five minutes at the beginning of the meeting in order to make some dramatic announcement. With the meaning of her behavior reframed and the attention placed on her, according to the terms of the therapist and Househead, she quickly declined comment and stopped her dramatic pronouncements.

As a result of these interventions the staff found the client much more pleasant to be around, much less demanding and thereby more willing to respond to her emotional needs. This case also demonstrated the necessary interaction between house staff and the family therapist in order for effective change to occur. A dysfunctional triad of house staff, client and family therapist was avoided. In addition, the case provided an opportunity for the house staff to positively connote and reframe the client's behavior and to prescribe symptomatic behavior.

Certainly a major difference in the strategic/systemic approach of the VCA to change as compared to the more traditional approach to therapy is that the therapeutic techniques of paradox, reframing, illusion of alternatives, positive connotation, can be readily learned and applied by nontherapists. The teaching of these clinical techniques to nonclinically trained staff must be done with care such that any one technique is not used inappropriately or out of context. Interestingly, the house staff reported that they often used paradox, illusion of alternatives, etc. without knowing their formal labels. Learning such techniques within a clinical context seemed to enhance the house staff's repertoire of skills and sense of empowerment. This approach to the youth care workers was received quite positively by the workers themselves and by management. One of the authors (Roberts) was invited back two years after she left the agency for the purpose of providing a similar training package for new house staff.

SUMMARY

In summary, four general areas need to be considered for the effective introduction of systems family therapy into a traditionally oriented organization:

1. Recognition that the agency is a system organized with a hierarchy and rules similar to a family. There is a homeostatic tendency in all systems. Therefore, entrance into such a system must be done so as to carefully consider the hierarchy and boundaries of that system and the context in which family therapy will be viewed by other staff.
2. Joining with the system is essential. The family therapist needs to avoid the pitfalls of symmetrical escalation and/or dysfunctional triadic relationships with other components within the agency. Oftentimes, taking a one-down position relative to another therapist or staff member can be of value in being able to demonstrate one's expertise in a nonthreatening way. In addition, such a one-down position can allow for an appreciation of another's skills.
3. Use of videotape presentations of family work in conjunction with ongoing training in systems theory and techniques in order to enhance staff skill and treatment repertoire.
4. Informing line staff, when appropriate, of possible responses to a particular family intervention so as to increase their involvement with the family work and reduce the possibility of sabotaging treatment.

These suggestions are not intended as mere techniques for the family therapist to gain power in the system but are intended to show respect for co-workers and provide a way to increase the system's flexibility in a productive manner. Family systems approach is applicable at a number of different levels within an agency. The systems therapist must be able to utilize a systems approach not only at the family level but at the level in which family work will occur in the agency.

REFERENCES

Bergman, J. (1980). The use of paradox in a community home for the chronically disturbed and retarded. *Family Process*, *19*, 65-71.

Fisch, R., Weakland, J., & Segal, L. (1983). *The tactics of change: Doing therapy briefly*. San Francisco: Jossey-Bass, Inc.

Guerin, P., & Pendagast, E. (1976). Evaluation of family system and genogram. In P. Guerin (ed.), *Family therapy theory and practice*. New York: Gardner Press.

Haley, J. (1976). *Problem solving therapy*. San Francisco: Jossey-Bass, Inc.

Held, B. (1982). Entering a mental health system: A strategic-systemic approach. *Journal of Strategic and Systemic Therapies*, *1*, 40-51.

Hoffman, L. (1981). *Foundations of family therapy*. New York: Basic Books, Inc.

Imber-Coppersmith, E. (1983). The place of family therapy in the homeostasis of larger systems. In M. Aronson & R. Wolberg (eds.), *Group & family therapy, 1982: An overview*. New York: Brunner/Mazel.

Jesse, E., & L'Abate, L. (1980). The use of paradox with children in an inpatient setting. *Family Process*, *19*, 59-64.

Pfeiffer, W. J., & Jones, J. E. (1970). *A handbook of structured experiences for human relations training* (Vols. I & II). Iowa City: University Associates Press.

Roberts, J. (1982). *Skill development in structural & strategic family therapy: Two models of live supervision*. Unpublished doctoral dissertation, Microfilm #8229598.

Selvini-Palazzoli, M., Boscolo, L., Cecchin, G., & Prata, G. (1978). *Paradox and counterparadox*. New York: Jason Aronson.

Selvini-Palazzoi, M., Boscolo, L., Cecchin, G., & Prata, G. (1980). Hypothesizing-circularity-neutrality: Three guidelines for the conduction of the sessions. *Family Process*, *19*, 3-12.

Spolin, V. (1963). *Improvisation for the theatre*. Evanston, IL: Northwestern University Press.

Tomm, K. (1982). The Milan approach to family therapy: A tentative report. In D. Freeman & B. Trute (eds.), *Treating families with special needs*. Ontario, Canada: Canadian Association of Social Workers.

Watzlawick, P., Weakland, J. H., & Fisch, R. (1974). *Change: Principles of problem formation and problem resolution*. New York: W. W. Norton & Co.

Weakland, J. H., Fisch, R., Watzlawick, P., & Godin, A. M. (1974). Brief therapy: Focused problem resolution. *Family Process*, *13*, 141-168.

PARENT TRAINING AND PREVENTION APPROACHES

Parent Training for Delinquency Prevention

Mark W. Fraser
J. David Hawkins
Matthew O. Howard

ABSTRACT. The use of consistent contingent child rearing practices by parents has been shown to increase family attachment and cohesion, and decrease delinquent behaviors among children. Research indicates that these practices can be successfully taught through parent training. This paper describes the components of parent training, reviews implementation issues, and discusses research findings and implications. Practical problems associated with this

Mark W. Fraser is affiliated with the University of Utah School of Social Work, Salt Lake City, UT 84112; J. David Hawkins and Matthew O. Howard are affiliated with the University of Washington School of Social Work, JH-30, 4101 Fifteenth Avenue NE, Seattle, WA 98195. Prepared under grants from the National Institute for Juvenile Justice and Delinquency Prevention, U.S. Department of Justice, and the National Institute on Drug Abuse. Points of view or opinions in this document are those of the authors and do not necessarily represent official positions or policies of the U.S. Department of Justice or the National Institute on Drug Abuse.

approach that may limit its widespread use as a major delinquency prevention strategy are discussed. Areas for further research are identified.

Scholars have speculated on the relationship between the family and delinquent behavior for years. There is evidence to support the existence of a biological predisposition toward crime transmitted through families. There is also evidence that experiences in the family during the process of development contribute to delinquent behavior (Wilson & Herrnstein, 1985).

Researchers have found that family attachment variables have independent effects on delinquent behavior (Hirschi, 1969). It appears that the process of socialization in the family is involved in the etiology of delinquency and is a promising target for delinquency prevention activities.

Unfortunately, a number of delinquency prevention efforts targeted on youths and their families have failed to demonstrate effectiveness when subjected to rigorous evaluation (Berleman, 1980). The social casework and counseling model of individual and family interventions tested in the Cambridge-Somerville Youth Study failed to prevent officially recorded delinquent offenses (Powers & Witmer, 1951). The child guidance model tested by the New York City Youth Board was based on the Glueck's Social Prediction Table (Craig & Furst, 1965), reflecting the view that disorganized family life was the source of delinquent behavior. It also failed to prevent officially recorded delinquency (Berleman, 1980). Similarly, Washington D.C.'s Maximum Benefits Project, a social casework-oriented model based on the Glueck's Prediction Table, failed to prevent delinquency (Berleman, 1980). Apparently, these family counseling and casework approaches to delinquency prevention did not adequately address the family variables important in the etiology of delinquency.

In contrast, encouraging results have been obtained in several small family-focused research projects which attempted to alter family practices related to delinquent behavior (Alexander & Parsons, 1973; Klein et al., 1977; Patterson, 1974b, 1982). In these projects, parents were engaged actively in structured educational programs which trained them in specific skills. This paper reviews this educational approach to family-focused delinquency prevention. The approach is cognitive behavioral parent training.

The paper presents a framework for assessing parent training, reviews the history and theoretical bases for the approach, describes its components, and reviews implementation and practice issues associated with parent training. Finally, research results and studies needed are discussed from a delinquency prevention perspective.

A FRAMEWORK FOR PARENT TRAINING

Given the gloomy results of many past efforts, on what foundation can family-oriented prevention programs be based? Hawkins and Weis (1985) have proposed a model of delinquency as a basis for empirically supportable intervention. Their social development approach is a synthesis of social control theory and social learning theory. The model identifies the family, school, and peer group as major social units in which youths develop and hypothesizes that a child's attachment to conventional actors within these social units is associated with an absence of delinquent behavior. It suggests that the greater the degree of attachment to prosocial others, the lower the probability of delinquency. The model hypothesizes that the formation of attachment in a social unit is contingent upon three factors: (1) the extent to which opportunities for participation in the social unit are available to the individual; (2) the skills which the individual uses in participating in the social unit whether in completing tasks, solving problems, or interacting with others; and (3) the reinforcements (both positive and negative) that are provided through the social unit for behaviors that conform to the unit's expectations.

From a developmental perspective, establishing a social bond to the family is extremely important. Social bonding to the family provides a base of support from which the child can develop bonds to other social units encountered later in the process of social development.

The social development perspective provides a provisional set of criteria for assessing the promise of family-oriented delinquency prevention approaches. Interventions in the family should increase *opportunities* for the child's involvement in prosocial interactions and activities, increase the child's *skills* for participation in the family and beyond, and insure the frequency and consistency of *rewards* for prosocial participation by the child. Where this is achieved, a social bond can be expected to develop between the child and his or her family. This bond of attachment should inhibit delinquent behavior. Thus, parent training may reduce juvenile crime by increasing parents' skills to create opportunities for involvement and interaction in the family for their children, to set clear expectations for their children, and to practice consistent and contingent family management.

HISTORY OF PARENT TRAINING

Parent training was advanced significantly in the 1960s when behavioral therapists sought to extend clinical practices into the home. Wahler (1969a), Patterson et al. (1967b), Hawkins et al. (1966), and others argued that clinically significant changes were of practical importance only if parents were able to influence their child's behavior in the home, independent of direct clinical control. In a series of small studies, they developed interventions to achieve this goal and observational measures to test changes in clinic and home settings (Tighe & Elliott, 1968). Concomitantly, social workers attempting to teach child management skills to groups of low-income parents were achieving moderate success (Wittes & Radin, 1971). The advances in the last 15 years have made parent training an interventive tool with potential for delinquency prevention.

Research has demonstrated that parents can be trained to modify the behavior of their children (Loeber & Stouthamer-Loeber, 1985). Using single subject, multiple baseline or reversal designs, and no treatment control, placebo control, and alternate treatment control group designs, numerous studies have demonstrated the effectiveness of parent training (Briar & Conte, 1978). Parent training has been shown to increase school achievement and decrease stealing, fighting, and disruptive behaviors (Patterson, 1974a, 1974b). While there have been some failures, on balance the evidence indicates that the intervention is effective when it is applied to parents of children under the age of 15.

THE INTERVENTION

Parent training is rooted in behavior therapy and is guided by seven basic principles (Rimm & Masters, 1978):

1. Behavior itself is important. No underlying, psychological "roots" of behavior need be addressed.
2. Delinquent behaviors of children are learned.[1]
3. Anyone can learn new skills. Principles of learning theory can be effectively applied to minimize undesirable behavior.[2]
4. Undesirable behaviors can be partitioned into smaller, manageable component behaviors.
5. Delinquent behavior arises in specific interactions in response to situational social stimuli which can be altered.
6. Current, observable problems are most amenable to intervention.
7. Observing and recording results rewards family members' participation, leading to sustained involvement in the intervention.

Parent training arose from the attempts of behavior therapists to influence the natural environment by engaging parents in behavior management roles in the household. Parent training builds the capacity of family members to solve problems by providing parents and children with specific skills and a conflict reduction plan. It focuses on concrete events, distinct skills, and repeated practice. Parent training combines knowledge building with skill development in a supportive environment, often a parents' group. Typically, trainers use lectures, reading assignments, or videotapes to provide instruction in skills, followed by demonstration, modeling, and supervised practice to insure skill acquisition at the level of application. Although the mixture of emphases on knowledge, skill, and practice varies, the use of a group format is reasonably consistent. The elements of parent training are reviewed in greater detail below.

Knowledge Building

Many programs try to create a common denominator of basic knowledge among participants. Some do this by requiring reading prior to the beginning of parent training. In their work with parents of aggressive or stealing boys, Reid and Patterson (1976) attempted to establish a language base by requiring parents to pass a test on basic social learning concepts. Fleischman (1981) used didactic instruction and reading of a programmed text describing application of social learning principles to child rearing, to ensure a common conceptual orientation in parents of boys with conduct disorders. The parent training approach assumes the importance of consistent, mild rewards and punishments. Those parents who respond inconsistently to the same act or who tend to use harsh punishments may have difficulty valuing and implementing the approach. Reading assignments and tests are designed to reduce this possibility by emphasizing that child management is a complex task requiring consistency and moderation. The assignments seek to establish both a common language and a common value system. These may also be established by lectures or videotapes.

Skill Development

The skills taught in parenting training include, but are not limited to, behavioral observation, contract negotiation, and contingency administration. Often, these are modeled by the trainer and then practiced by parents in small groups.

Use of Contingencies

When rewards and punishments are given for a particular behavior, they are called contingencies. Parent training assumes that the perception of desired and undesired responses for a given behavior will influence the frequency of that behavior. Those behaviors which are rewarded are likely to increase and those which are punished or ignored are likely to decrease. Children and parents come to anticipate desirable or undesirable consequences for behavior, and these predicted results guide subsequent actions. Of course, rewards and punishments vary in their potential to influence behavior. In the 1960s, behavioral training for parents focused largely upon extinction and conditioning. Punishment was thought to be ineffective and to have deleterious side effects. However, the technique of rewarding children for prosocial behaviors and ignoring antisocial behaviors did not prove to be as effective as treatment which included both the use of mild punishment for undesirable behavior and rewards for desirable behavior (Patterson & Fleischman, 1979). In two small studies, Wahler (1969b) and Patterson et al. (1967b) demonstrated the successful use of both positive and negative rewards delivered in the form of a contingency contract. The more empirically grounded parenting approaches are rooted in the use of this technique.

Verbal or Written Contracts

The contingency contract is a basic tool of parent training. It specifies desirable and undesirable behaviors for which rewards and punishments will be given to the child by the parent. The purpose of the contract is to make concrete, objective, and explicit what is to be done. Consequently, the contract contains statements defining desired and undesired behaviors, privileges, rewards (privileges which are to be earned), bonuses (for exemplary performance), sanctions (to indicate in advance how parents will act in the case of undesired behaviors), and a monitoring method. To the extent that it prescribes behavior for parents and clarifies desired behavior for the child, the contract is a useful tool. It is, however, time-consuming and somewhat cumbersome, and in a follow-up study, Wittes and Radin (1971) found that many parents had discarded its use. They reported continued contingent use of rewards and punishments for selected behaviors, and this may be the ultimate implementation goal in parent training.

Rewards

A contingency contract includes a schedule of rewards and punishments for specific behaviors. Rewards are given to encourage repetition of a desirable behavior and they can be tangible or social, but, in practice, most are social. Parents may give praise, a warm smile, or a hug in response to desirable behavior. Rewards may vary from a word of recognition for a job well done to the accumulation of points which can be exchanged by the child for desired goods or services. The size and nature of rewards offered usually is related to the difficulty of the objective, the child's orientation toward tangible and social reinforcements and the parents' comfort with the use of various rewards.

Mild Punishment

Physical punishment is never considered mild and is not advocated by most parent trainers. However, parent trainers have developed responses for dealing with undesired behaviors.

Time out. When isolation or ignoring are used as mild punishments for specific behaviors, they are called time out. To be effective, time out must be unstimulating and of limited duration. O'Dell et al. (1980) suggest the following practice guidelines for its use:

a. Designate a spot or room as the time out center. It should have no toys, comic books, record players, or other stimulating distractions.
b. Set a standard time limit, such as five minutes, for punishment.
c. After misbehavior, lead the child to the time out center.
d. If the child comes out early, lead him/her back.
e. If the child refuses, do not force compliance. Use an additional consequence for noncompliance, such as loss of TV privileges for one evening.

Time out appears to be more effective when parents use clear, precise language. Roberts et al. (1978) investigated the effects of using specific commands with noncompliant 3 to 7-year-old children (N = 27). In contrast to a no treatment control group and a placebo group which used an active listening technique adapted from parent effectiveness training (Gordon, 1970), groups using a specific command style were observed to have significantly higher rates of child compliance.[3] The compliance rate for the group using time out plus the command style was superior to that of a group using only the command style. This study implies that mild punishment in the form of time out combined with training in communication skills is a more effective intervention for managing children's behavior than is communication skills training alone. Martin (1977) found training in both communication and contingency management skills, including time out, to result in significant reductions in weekly parental estimates of children's misbehaviors. While parental self-reports of behavior change may be biased (Griest & Wells, 1983), this study suggests the promise of parent training in contingency management and communication skills for the treatment of childhood conduct disorders and predelinquent behaviors. Future research should aim at assessing the independent contributions of each approach to treatment outcome.

Freeze. In contrast to time out, an approach called the "freeze technique" was evaluated by Pinkston and Herbert-Jackson (1975). In this study, parents of severely handicapped children were taught to "freeze" for 15 seconds following the occurrence of undesirable targeted behavior. The single subject study (N = 2) showed reduced asocial behavior by children when parents used this ignoring technique in comparison with an attention-giving baseline. In this study, brief, almost stop-action, time outs were used to curb disruptive behavior. To date, little research has addressed the comparative effectiveness of isolation versus the freeze technique, but it does appear that there are several types of ignoring which can be used to negatively sanction undesired behavior.

Response cost. In parent training, the conditional loss of rewards or privileges is often used as a backup to ignoring techniques. When a child fails to comply with time out, for example, a privilege may be withdrawn (O'Dell et al., 1980). Such privileges may include allowance, TV time or dessert. When something already earned is taken away, it is called "response cost." Response cost punishment has been used to change a number of behaviors such as smoking (Elliott & Tighe, 1968) and school performance of developmentally disabled children (Arnold et al., 1976). As an interventive technique, it appears to be more compelling than time out because it clearly involves an undesirable consequence (O'Dell et al., 1977; Rimm & Masters, 1978). For parents and children who are enmeshed in coercive interactions, time out may be insufficient and the intervention may be expanded to include response costs.

RESEARCH FINDINGS

Methodologically, much of the existing research on parent training is characterized by poor sampling, small sample sizes, weak designs, and inadequate measurement (Briar & Conte, 1978). Exclusive reliance upon parent reports of change without home observation appears to be neither valid nor reliable (Eyeberg & Johnson, 1974; Griest & Wells, 1983). For this reason, many researchers have adopted observational measures. While some researchers have used random assignment to experimental and control conditions, few multiple group studies with adequate samples to allow confident conclusions have been reported. Exceptions are the recent controlled studies of Patterson and his associates (Patterson et al., 1982) which have shown reductions in aversive behaviors for children randomly assigned to experimental parent training when compared with children in control conditions.

Research over the past 15 years indicates that parents can be trained to change the behavior of their children in the home (Fleishman, 1981; Patterson & Reid, 1973) and, to a less substantiated degree, in the school (Patterson & Fleischman, 1979). Parents have been taught to negotiate contingency contracts which reward children for prosocial behaviors and which discourage undesired behaviors ranging from temper tantrums to stealing. In more than 65% of the published studies, significant improvements subsequent to treatment have been reported (Patterson & Fleischman, 1979). Moreover, some studies have reported increases in parent-child attachment and decreases in skill deficits, variables which are significantly associated with delinquency (Hirschi, 1969; Karoly & Rosenthal, 1977; Patterson & Reid, 1973). There are also indications that after parent training, expectations within the home become clearer and overall levels of conflict and confusion are reduced. Thus, parent training appears to affect variables associated with delinquency. It also has shown positive effects on such delinquent behaviors as stealing (Loeber & Stouthamer-Loeber, 1985). However, research has only begun to address the question of whether improvements in targeted child behaviors generalize to other settings and behaviors.

IMPLEMENTATION ISSUES AND RESEARCH QUESTIONS

While the basic elements of parent training have been systematized, a number of practical issues and research questions remain to be addressed. These are reviewed below.

Disproportionate Availability

Like many family-oriented prevention programs, parent training appears to be disproportionately available to white families. From a national survey of delinquency prevention programs, Hawkins and Salisbury (1983) report that the likelihood of providing family-oriented services decreases as the proportion of nonwhites served increases. Though no systematic survey of this issue has been undertaken with regard to parent training specifically, this exploratory survey suggests that agencies which provide parent training may be less likely to serve minorities than whites.

Attrition

A major problem confronted in all family therapies including parent training is attrition (Griest & Wells, 1983; Loeber & Stouthamer-Loeber, 1985). Patterson et al. (1982) report that 22% of the families they recruited dropped out before or during baseline observations. Two other studies at the Oregon Social Learning Center found that 43 and 32% of families in treatment terminated against therapist's advice or totally refused to comply with treatment requirements (Fleishman, 1981; Patterson, 1974b). Firestone et al. (1980) reported a 50% dropout rate with parents of children with conduct disorders, while Eyeberg and Johnson (1974) reported a loss of 45% of families with conduct disordered children. Attrition rates of this magnitude severely limit the generalizability of conclusions regarding the effectiveness of parent training. Participant dropout appears to be associated with the perception of the quality of the program, the appeal of the trainer, the trainer's attributes and expectations, the client's attributes and expectations, and situational or demographic characteristics (Shapiro, 1974). However, Patterson (1982), Reid and Patterson (1976), Weathers and Liberman (1975), and Wahler et al. (1979) report that disruption and disorganization of the social environment within and beyond the family also account for attrition. Since social and economic environmental factors such as poverty, family acrimony, poor housing, and high rates of community deviance also are associated with delinquency, the families which are most likely to drop out of parenting training may be those in which delinquent behavior is most likely to occur.

Delinquency-focused parent training programs have developed attrition reduction strategies. These have included a variety of social and tangible inducements, such as the provision of child care during training sessions, provision of free training materials, emphasis on building a group identity and financial rewards for attendance. Practitioners observe that positive group experiences are associated with regular attendance. Parents who contact other parents either informally or by design (e.g., in weekly parents' phone trees) appear more likely to participate (Gold, 1981). Fleischman and Szykula (1980) developed an aggressive recruitment and supportive services approach which decreased dropout among low-income AFDC and single parent families. Their approach included prompt follow-up of initial contact, home visits, *in vivo* training, evening meetings (at the family's convenience), written contracts, and concrete problem solving.

To reduce attrition, other clinicians have used financial incentives. Eyberg and Johnson (1974) randomly assigned parents of oppositional children to a deposit (fee deposited in advance) or training-free-of-charge condition. They found that the deposit significantly increased attendance and completion of homework assignments by participating parents. Similarly, Glogower and Sloop (1976) required a $25 deposit which was returned to parents only if good attendance was maintained throughout the training. Though he permitted some negotiation, Rose (1974) required a $10 deposit for AFDC and middle-income trainees, and Patterson et al. (1975) required a $10-$25 deposit against broken appointments. Using different techniques, Karoly and Rosenthal (1977) paid parents $5 for each meeting attended and Wittes and Radin (1971) gave parents toys and games for their children.

To test the effectiveness of "parenting salaries" on cooperation and attendance, Fleischman (1971) experimentally manipulated dollar amounts paid to parents-in-training while controlling for family income. Families were randomly assigned to a no payment group or to a group in which they received $1 for each day of compliance with the treatment plan. The results suggest that financial incentives increase attendance and cooperation, and reduce attrition among low-income, single parent families. However, Martin (1977) found that participation rates of middle-class families in parent training programs were unaffected by incentive payments. Parents were paid $10 at the beginning of a study examining the effectiveness of a short-term parent training program in treating childhood oppositional disorders, and $10 if they completed all assessment procedures at the end of the year. Payments were not made the second year of the project, and parental participation rates were unaffected. The modest payments made by Martin (1977), and the fact that the majority of the families he studied were middle-class, may account for his failure to find effects of incentive payments.

Use of Siblings and Peers as Adjunctive Therapists

During adolescence, the importance of peers in influencing behavior increases (Elliott et al., 1985; Jessor & Jessor, 1977). Thus, the use of peers and siblings as adjuncts in parent training may be warranted. Two methods to expand the power of parent training interventions by involving peers or siblings appear promising.

The first is the inclusion of a sibling as an adjunctive therapist. The "helper therapy principle" (Reisman, 1965) suggests that the probability of change in the subject and in the helper is increased when siblings are included in treatment as helpers. The use of siblings as helpers may be particularly powerful as a delinquency prevention strategy given Taplin and Reid's (1977) findings of high rates of deviant behavior among nontargeted children in families with aggressive or stealing children.

Lavigueur (1976) investigated the use of siblings as helpers in a child management program using positive reinforcement, extinction, and time out techniques. In a black, working-class family and a white, upper middle-class family (N = 2), parents and siblings of oppositional children were trained to positively respond to desired behaviors and to ignore oppositional behavior. The children referred for treatment were described as rude, noncompliant, and demanding, but neither child was delinquent. In the first family, the referred child was 12 years old and her ten-year-old sister was trained as a helper. In the second, the target child was nine and his ten-year-old brother was trained. The results suggest that when siblings have a history of triggering the deviant behaviors of an identified child, the inappropriate behaviors of both can be reduced by recruitment of the sibling as an adjunctive therapist. To date, the use of siblings in adjunctive roles has not been tested in controlled studies though it is a logical extension of parent training.

A second promising strategy is the recruitment of peers as adjunctive therapists. This approach has been shown to increase children's success experiences in school (Shaver & Nuhn, 1971), but has been little reported in the parent training literature. Trovato and Bucher (1980) applied the principle of parent and peer involvement to remedial tutoring. Members of triads matched on reading ability were randomly assigned to conditions of peer tutoring (N = 23), peer tutoring with home-based rewards (N = 23), or no special treatment (N = 23). The investigators found that both peer tutoring programs significantly increased reading achievement in comparison with the control group which received a normal school program. Moreover, gains in the home-based rewards/peer tutoring group were twice as great as in the peer tutoring only group. This result suggests that peers might also be successfully involved in supporting parents in behavior management programs.

Length of Training

There is no agreement as to the appropriate length of parent training. While from an implementation perspective it is desirable to standardize the amount of training, families appear to respond differently to fixed amounts of treatment. In recognition of this, Patterson et al. (1975) adopted a "fade out" treatment design. After approximately ten two-hour training sessions, follow-up sessions were scheduled with decreasing frequency. The length of "fade out" was based upon the speed of skill acquisition by parents. While an average family required 31.2 hours of treatment in Patterson's program, some low-income, crisis-prone families required twice that (Patterson, 1974b). In a replication of Patterson's (1974b) study, Fleischman (1981) standardized the delivery of treatment by constructing a therapy manual which detailed material to be covered at each treatment session. There was a sizable reduction in the number of hours clients spent in treatment (13.7 vs. 31.2). The interventions produced comparable reductions in total aversive childhood behaviors from baseline to posttreatment (43% in Patterson, 1974b; 42% in Fleischman, 1981). Martin found significant reductions in maternal reports of mother-child conflict with total therapy contact limited to ten hours (Martin, 1977). Similar results are reported by Baum and Forehand (1981) and Johnson and Christensen (1975), although other time-limited interventions without flexible "fade out" have failed to produce enduring changes (Eyeberg & Johnson, 1974; Patterson, 1982; Weathers & Liberman, 1975). Variability in rates of parental skill acquisition may limit the utility of a fixed length intervention, while economic considerations may limit widespread adoption of an open-ended approach. This issue merits further research.

Group or Individual Training

While most parent trainers use group instruction, little research has compared this method against the training of individual parents. Group training is less costly than individual training and may offer other benefits. For example, Oei and Jackson (1980) found a social skills intervention more effective in reducing abusive alcohol consumption, when administered in group rather than individual settings. They explained their results by referring to the opportunities for behavioral rehearsal and modeling provided in group settings. Wahler et al. (1979) have found that isolation in the community is associated with inconsistent and abusive child rearing practices. Griest and Wells (1983) reviewed a number of studies that found "insular" mothers to persist in coercive parent-child interactions more than twice as long as noninsular mothers. Families embedded in informal social networks appear to have access to many helping resources in times of stress, while isolated families lack problem-solving resources and tend to receive help only when problems are more severe. Parent training in groups which attend to the development of group cohesion may serve to increase family connections, thereby increasing the probability of successful child rearing.

Several clinicians have incorporated individual training in a group format. Wahler et al. (1979), Patterson (1979), and Fleischman and Szykula (1980) have used both individual and group methods. Patterson, Szykula, and Fleischman supplemented group training with individual sessions. In fact, much of their recent work has been individually focused; one family is seen at a time with families that progress slowly being seen more often. This reactive use of individual sessions differs from Wahler's approach. He reports success using a treatment method in which individual families engage in structured problem solving before entering parent training groups.

Training Costs

To address questions of cost-effectiveness, Christensen et al. (1980) compared group and individual conditions with self-instruction using self-help training materials (bibliotherapy). On a number of measures, both the individual and group conditions were essentially equivalent, and both showed significantly better outcomes than bibliotherapy. Since the individualized program required over 11 hours of professional time per family, and the group training five hours, the group approach was regarded as most cost-effective.

The issue of cost raises questions regarding the use of professionals in parent training. Patterson (1982), in describing his unsuccessful parenting groups, has attributed failure to the use of "time-limited treatment procedures (that) were carried out by graduate student therapists" (p. 305). Yet, research has not specified what it is that professionals do that facilitates behavioral change. In comparing graduate student trainees with experienced professionals, Fleischman (1979) found that both correctly presented the training technology, but that the latter were more animated and warm.

Since parent training has generally been shown to be effective (Loeber & Stouthamer-Loeber, 1985), it is noteworthy that many failures appear to be associated with the use of less experienced, less costly therapists. But this issue is worthy of more investigation.

Supplementing Parent Training with Problem Solving, Negotiation Skills, and Communication Skills Training

Since parent training usually includes the negotiation of contingency contracts with children, some trainers have included training in negotiation and problem-solving processes (Weathers & Liberman, 1975).

Robin and his associates (1981) hypothesize that parent-adolescent conflict arises from the failure of family members to negotiate mutually acceptable solutions to daily problems, viewing conflict as a result of skill deficits and inappropriate attitudinal responses leading to reciprocally punishing transactions. In their early work (Robin et al., 1977), parent-adolescent dyads (N = 24) matched on SES and communication skills were randomly assigned to training or a waiting-list control. In five one-hour sessions, a problem-solving/communications skills model was taught: (1) define a problem; (2) list alternative solutions; (3) evaluate each alternative; and (4) plan the implementation of one solution. After training, the experimental trainees were significantly more skillful in utilizing problem solving and negotiation skills in both real and hypothetical situations. However, negative in-home behaviors (commands, threats, expletives) were not affected. Given Patterson and Stouthamer-Loeber's (1984) recent failure to find an association between problem-solving practices in the family and self or officially reported delinquency, it is not clear that problem-solving skills training alone will alter variables associated with delinquency. Patterson and Stouthamer-Loeber (1984) found that parental monitoring of youth whereabouts and disciplinary practices did explain substantial amounts of variance in delinquency. They suggest that certain family management practices may be salient in the development of prosocial behaviors, while others are central to the fostering of antisocial conduct. It is possible that problem solving in the family is important in the development of prosocial relations, but is not directly related to antisocial conduct.

To date, few controlled studies of the combined use of contingency contracting and communications training have been reported. Alexander and Parsons (1973) varied use of these methods across subjects in their evaluation of a complex parent training intervention. During a six- to 18-month follow-up, juvenile court referral rates for children in a combined contingency contracting/communication skills condition were roughly half those of children in comparison and control groups. The parent training treatment significantly altered patterns of communication within participating families and appears to have reduced subsequent offenses in the high-risk sample (Alexander & Parsons, 1980).

A combined problem-solving and communications-focused approach to family intervention is Parent Effectiveness Training (P.E.T.) (Gordon, 1970). P.E.T. does not make use of contingency management, but is based on a communications model which asserts that inadequate listening and expressive skills impair family members' abilities to engage in mutual problem solving, and that unresolved problems lead to acts of deviance (Gordon, 1970).

P.E.T. consists of training in structured problem solving, active listening, and the giving of "I-messages," (e.g., "I feel angry when you don't put gas in the car."). Several controlled studies indicate that P.E.T. improves parents' acceptance and understanding of their children (e.g., Williams & Sanders, 1974). Miles (1974) reports significant reductions in teacher ratings of school problem behaviors of children whose parents received P.E.T. This generalization across settings is particularly promising since the teacher raters in Miles' study were randomly selected and blind to the condition of the students' rated. However, most research on P.E.T. is based upon parent and child self-report data. Few studies report behavioral change and few report follow-up. Where follow-up data are available, P.E.T. has not demonstrated effectiveness over time (Janiak, 1975).

Communications training used as an adjunct to contingency management in parent training programs should be subjected to additional controlled study.

The Use of Print and Video

From a prevention perspective, it would be desirable to provide parent training to out-of-clinic populations through the use of film, video, texts, and other media. Self-administered materials are considerably less expensive than professionally supervised training. Some advice packages for parents in various forms of media have produced desirable results when the advice was limited to specific situations (O'Dell et al., 1979).

For example, Clark et al. (1976) found in a community survey that the disruptive behavior of children while on family shopping trips was a problem for which many parents were seeking a solution. The investigators constructed a self-administered program with two instructional components:

1. Response Cost Technique. Each child was given 50¢ allowance for a shopping trip. Every time the child engaged in disruptive or oppositional behavior, 5¢ was subtracted from the allotment. Children could spend what was left of the allowance at the end of the trip.
2. Enhancement. Parents were instructed to engage the child in conversation about shopping (and other topics) as a way of increasing the child's involvement in the activity.

A four-part, "Parent Advice Packet for Family Shopping Trips" was compiled. Part 1 described both the techniques in text form; Part 11 consisted of self-administered quizzes; Part III contained tally sheets, shopping lists, and self-feedback questions; and Part IV gave examples of conversations explaining the experiment to children.

To test these packets, four mothers and their children from lower middle and middle-class backgrounds were paid $4 for each shopping trip and received a $20 bonus if all appointments were kept. Packets were given to mothers in their homes, and, for a period of four days, families practiced shopping trips. Observers rated change in both parent and child behavior. In all four families, the intervention appeared to reduce the disruptive behavior of children, to increase social/educational interaction between children and parents, and to decrease the punitive behavior of parents.

In a replication study with six mothers and their children using the same materials, similar results were found. It should be noted that in both studies, trainers intervened to test parents' knowledge prior to the practice phase. If parents failed quizzes, they were instructed to reread the programmed text. Thus, the intervention was supervised and payment of a fee introduced an external incentive.

McMahon and Forehand (1978) addressed these issues in an attempt to evaluate the effectiveness of a brochure designed to teach mothers to correct their children's inappropriate mealtime behaviors. Following baseline data collection, three middle-class, college-educated mothers of pre-school age children were given a two and one-half page brochure which explained the use of differential attention and time out. The experimenters made no attempt to clarify the brochure or to ascertain the mothers' understanding of the material. Monetary incentives for participation were not provided. During mealtime, observers recorded parental use of contingencies and the child's mealtime behavior. All three mothers demonstrated increased use of rewards, and substantial decreases in children's inappropriate mealtime behaviors were found. Six weeks afterwards, these changes had eroded but remained improved over baseline levels.

The use of video to demonstrate appropriate parent behavior in a variety of parenting situations, also has yielded promising results. Using video plus group discussion, Webster-Stratton (1981) reported significant decreases in mothers' leadtaking, dominating, and nonacceptance behaviors at the end of treatment and at a six-week follow-up. This investigation involved no control group and used middle-class, college-educated subjects. The findings suggest that video may offer an inexpensive mode for training some parents.

While books, pamphlets and videotapes may offer a low-cost alternative to parent training by professionals, there are indications that partial understanding and misunderstanding may result from the use of such materials. These misunderstandings can lead to serious errors in the use of contingencies. Christensen et al. (1980) reported that five of ten self-trained parents who read *Living With Children* (Patterson & Gullion, 1971) misapplied behavioral techniques. Three used punishment excessively. As noted earlier, this experimental study found that group and individual training approaches were superior to bibliotherapy alone. While bibliotherapy may work for a portion of the parents who request assistance with child rearing, until research clarifies who will benefit and who will not, books, pamphlets and videotapes may be best used to supplement rather than supplant parenting training (O'Dell et al., 1979). The use of such material as a supplement in parent training is worthy of more rigorous research.

Generalization of Parent Skills to Deal with Other Child Behaviors

Typically, in parent training, parents choose one or two child behaviors upon which to focus. A critical question in terms of delinquency prevention is whether parents who learn the skills to change one or two child behaviors apply their skills to behaviors which occur in other settings and times. Griest and Wells (1983) report that a parent training intervention that successfully reduced identified problem behaviors in children, also reduced rates of nontarget behaviors, including excessive crying and aggressiveness. These results suggest that parent training may have broad preventive potential. However, parents with more disruptive children are least motivated in training (Patterson, 1982). Though these parents can be trained to modify their children's targeted delinquent behaviors (Reid et al., 1980), long-term follow-up shows that many children of trained parents fail to desist from subsequent illegal acts after parent training is discontinued (Moore et al., 1979).

Several attempts to broaden the application of parenting skills have involved the teaching of principles of social learning. The addition of instruction in social learning principles to standard parent training packages, has been shown to produce stronger treatment effects than parent training alone (Glogower & Sloop, 1976). McMahon et al. (1981) found that children in a social learning instruction group were more compliant and were perceived by their parents as better adjusted at three-month follow-up, than children in a parent training only group.

To address the generalization issue, Sanders and Glynn (1981) tested a self-management intervention against a more standard skills training approach. They hypothesized that different parenting settings in the home and community provide different cues to initiate appropriate parental intervention. Consequently, they devised a self-management approach in which parents planned interventions for different environments. This augmented a standard program of in-home parent training. Parents in the self-management training condition were found to use their new parenting skills in a cross-section of out-of-home settings. These results suggest that both anticipatory planning techniques and teaching principles of social learning may help to generalize parent skills and increase the potential for preventing delinquency. However, more rigorous evaluation with larger samples is required to assess the nature and extent of effects of such supplementary training seeking to generalize parent skills.

Generalization of Children's Behavior Changes to Nontargeted Behaviors

In a closely related area, researchers have studied the extent to which changes in targeted child behaviors are associated with changes in other, nontargeted behaviors. Wahler et al. (1979) documented changes in such nontargeted behaviors as bedwetting and stuttering, and Patterson (1974b) reported near significant reductions in nontargeted behaviors. However, more controlled studies using observational data and large samples are needed to document possible changes in nontargeted child behaviors as a result of parent training.

Generalization of Effects to Other Children in the Family

If parent training changes what parents do, leading to better family communication, greater clarity and consistency of family norms, better family management practices, and greater parent and child attachment, it should reduce the likelihood of delinquency among all children in the family. In a follow-up of a parent training intervention (Parsons & Alexander, 1973), Klein et al. (1977) found reductions in the number of court referrals of siblings of targeted children whose parents participated in a skills training program. The generalization of treatment effects to other children in the family is an important finding. In this research, however, therapists' skill levels varied greatly, and the experimental and control treatments were delivered in different settings. This leaves open the possibility of a therapist by setting interaction in which the combination of setting and therapist influenced outcomes.

In a separate investigation of generalization to siblings, Arnold et al. (1975) studied 55 siblings of 27 "predelinquents" whose parents received parent training. Significant reductions in observed deviant behavior of siblings were found at the end of treatment and in a six-month follow-up. Biased attrition precluded testing at 12 months, but the results are promising.

Unfortunately, no measures of parent behavior are linked to the measures of sibling behavior in these studies. However, evidence of parental generalization of newly learned skills to siblings of the targeted child is provided by Humphreys et al. (1978), who found reductions in the rates of oppositional behaviors of nontargeted siblings. Reductions in sibling noncompliant behaviors were systematically related to changes in parental behavior attributable to parent training. While the results of these investigations are promising, the relationship between parent training and reductions in the levels of delinquency of nontargeted children in the family deserves further experimental study.

Durability of Effects

The most promising support for the durability of the effects of time-limited parent and family training on delinquent youth is reported by Alexander and Parsons (1973) and Klein et al. (1977). Diverted from the juvenile court to a child development center, 88 youths from primarily white, middle-class families were randomly assigned to family training, client-centered counseling, "dynamic" counseling, or a no treatment control. At the end of treatment, offenders and their families who received family training were shown to differ significantly from the control and comparison groups on a number of communications variables. During a follow-up period ranging from six to 18 months, the offenders in the family training condition had one-third to one-half as many court referrals as those in the other groups. Similar results appear to have been found in another parent training project (Berkowitz & Hazlewood, 1973).

While sample size is not indicated, this project randomly assigned court referred youths and their families to a behavioral treatment group using the "Simplified Analytical Methods of Behavior Systemization" (SAMBS) technique or no treatment control. At three, six, and 12 months following the ten two-hour SAMBS sessions, youths of the experimental group were found to have significantly lower rearrest rates.

Several studies also document effects lasting up to one year on less serious outcome measures such as fighting, whining, crying, and other forms of disruptive behavior which do not involve criminal activity (Patterson, 1974b; Patterson & Fleischman, 1979). However, only two document effects lasting more than a year. Baum and Forehand (1981) reported the maintenance of significant differences in parent and child behavior at periods ranging from one to more than four years after treatment. Strain et al. (1982) conducted a long-term follow-up (three to nine years) of 40 children who had exhibited severe tantrums, physical aggression toward parents, and other oppositional behaviors between the ages of three and five. At follow-up, no differences between randomly selected classroom peers and treated subjects were observed on school and home-based measures of compliant behavior suggesting long-term improvements in the behavior of oppositional children. Moreover, parent behavior in the home reflected the behavior management training received several years before. However, the absence of randomization to experimental and control conditions in this study makes regression to the mean and maturation plausible rival hypotheses to the authors' conclusion that parent training effected long-term reductions in childhood oppositional behaviors. Nevertheless, these findings suggest the possible promise of the use of parenting training as a preventive intervention seeking to increase parents' skills to inhibit their children's antisocial behaviors.

Applying Parent Training to High-Risk Populations

Moderate family stability appears to be a prerequisite for successful parent training (Wahler et al., 1979). Weathers and Liberman (1975) attempted to treat 28 multiple offense, male and female probationers between the ages of 14 and 17 in Ventura County, California. Using a short-term behavioral family intervention which included contingency contracting and negotiation skills training, they hoped to measure verbal abusiveness, curfew compliance, performance of chores, school achievement, and court referrals. Of the 28 families involved, 12 dropped out after the first home visit. Eight finished the baseline data collection, and only six completed the treatment and a three-month follow-up. Pre-post test differences for the six families who completed were not significant on any of the variables measured. The experience led the researchers to note:

> (In work with families) decimated by divorce, crime, drug abuse, inadequate communications/negotiation skills, the introduction of a contingency contract is worth about as much as the paper it's printed on. Consistent use of contingencies of reinforcement directed toward positive behavioral goals may be impossible to achieve in such families without some massive intervention that is currently not ethically acceptable or financially supportable by society.

Parents' interest in and ability to provide rewards and punishment in a consistent, contingent manner appear to be related to the stability of their social environment. Concurring with Weathers and Liberman, Patterson and Fleischman (1979) report that some low-income families have required "over 100 hours of treatment, and even then are a dubious success." Parent training failures with low-income families led Wahler (1980) to investigate environmental factors associated with successful and unsuccessful outcomes in parent training. He suggested that families "entrapped" by poverty, low education, unemployment, and hostile or indifferent intrafamily interactions cannot fulfill the demands placed upon them by society. For such families, consistent parenting may be a lower priority than the provision of food, shelter, and safety. These families do not appear to have the resources to provide consistent and powerful reinforcement to counteract the influence of other environmental forces such as the adolescent peer group (Wahler, 1980). It may be unrealistic to expect them to act consistently in the management of children (Patterson & Reid, 1973). At present, it appears that time-limited parent training is not likely to succeed with families plagued by crises, illness, unemployment, and poverty. So too, it appears less likely to succeed when parents are, themselves not bothered by, or are committed to, antisocial or illegal behaviors (Patterson, 1982). Unfortunately, these are families whose children are at great risk of serious delinquency (Elliott & Ageton, 1980).

For such high-risk families, a more concentrated, ongoing family-focused intervention may hold promise. With AFDC families, Fleischman and Szykula (1980) have demonstrated success with an approach incorporating both parent training and supportive problem solving. Patterson and his colleagues (1982) have shown that over a three-year period, arrests were significantly lower for children of parents in a treatment group which continued without termination than for children of parents randomly assigned to a group which received time-limited training. These results are encouraging and suggest that parent training may hold promise when implemented as part of a broader or more intensive program.

CONCLUSION

The family environment contributes both directly and indirectly to delinquent behavior (Bahr, 1979). Weak attachments to family members and family normlessness are both contributors (Hirschi, 1969). It appears that the use of consistent and contingent child rearing practices by parents can increase family attachment and cohesion, and decrease disruptive and delinquent behaviors among children. Further, a number of studies indicate that these practices can be successfully taught through parent training (Loeber & Stouthamer-Loeber, 1985). Thus, parent training holds promise as an approach to preventing delinquency.

Unfortunately, however, the extent of this promise is not fully known. Research on the generalization of parenting skills to other target behaviors and to other children in the family is needed as is research on generalization of behavioral change in children following parenting training. Additionally, research on the durability of effects of parenting training is needed before parent training's potential for preventing delinquency is known.

Further, a number of practical problems appear to be associated with the implementation of parent training. These may severely limit its broad application as a major delinquency prevention strategy. Among the most serious of these are problems encountered in recruiting and maintaining low-income families and families experiencing other types of disruption such as divorce or separation, social isolation, loss of a job, or health difficulties. Reliable methods for overcoming recruitment and attrition problems with such families must be demonstrated if the approach is to have widespread utility.

Finally, characteristics of family members themselves, such as drug abuse, excessive alcohol use or limited communication skills, may limit the ability of some families to use the practices taught in parenting classes. Families differ in many ways. One of these may be the extent to which members will learn and use the specific skills offered in parent training. This issue remains to be further investigated before the breadth of parent training's potential for preventing delinquency can be fully determined.

NOTES

1. Behavioral therapists do not claim that *all* behavior results from learning. Some investigators have argued that specific central nervous system dysfunctions may impair the learning of prosocial behaviors (Herrnstein, 1977).
2. However the ability to learn may be partially mediated by the attachment to significant others and the degree to which labels (e.g., "delinquent") limit others' expectations for change.
3. This command style was broken into three components:
    a. Clearly specify contingencies.
    b. Make a single command, e.g., "Do not throw that."
    c. Wait five seconds after giving the command before initiating a reinforcement (giving the child time to think about the desired and undesired consequences, make a choice, etc.).

REFERENCES

Alexander, J. F., & Parsons, B. V. (1973). Short-term behavioral intervention with delinquent families: Impact on family process and recidivism. *Journal of Abnormal Psychology*, *81*(3), 219-225.

Alexander, J. F., & Parsons, B. V. (1980). *Functional family therapy*. Monterey: Brooks/Cole.

Arnold, S. C., Forehand, R., & Sturgis, E. T. (1976). Effects of a response cost procedure on the academic performance of retarded students. *Journal of Behavior Therapy and Experimental Psychiatry*, 7, 191-192.

Arnold, J. E., Levine, A. G., & Patterson, G. R. (1975). Changes in sibling behavior following family intervention. *Journal of Consulting and Clinical Psychology*, *43*, 683-688.

Bahr, S. J. (1979). Family determinants and effects of deviance. In W. R. Burr, R. Hill, F. I. Nye, & I. L. Reiss (Eds.), *Contemporary theories about the family* (pp. 615-643). New York: The Free Press.

Baum, C., & Forehand, R. (1981). Long term follow-up assessment of parent training by use of multiple outcome measures. *Behavior Therapy*, *12*(5), 643-652.

Berkowitz, F. J., & Hazlewood, R. A. (1973). *Delinquency control through parent education. Evaluation of crime control programs in California: A review.* Sacramento, CA: California Council on Criminal Justice, pp. 27-30.

Berleman, W. C. (1980). Juvenile delinquency prevention experiments: A review and analysis. National Institute for Juvenile Justice and Delinquency Prevention, Office of Juvenile Justice and Delinquency Prevention, Law Enforcement Assistance Administration, U.S. Department of Justice. Washington, DC: U.S. Government Printing Office.

Briar, S., & Conte, J. R. (1978). Families. In H. S. Mass (Ed.), *Social service research: Reviews of studies* (pp. 9-38). Washington, DC: National Association of Social Workers.

Christensen, A., Johnson, S. M., Phillips, S., & Glasgow, R. E. (1980). Cost effectiveness in behavioral family therapy. *Behavior Therapy*, *11*, 208-226.

Clark, H. B., Risley, T. R., & Cataldo, M. F. (1976). Behavioral technology for the normal middle-class family. In E. J. Mash, L. A. Hamerlynck, & L. C. Handy (Eds.), *Behavior modification and families*. New York: Brunner/Mazel.

Craig, M. M., & Furst, P. W. (1965). What happens after treatment? A study of potentially delinquent boys. *Social Service Review*, *39*(2), 165-171.

Elliott, D. S., & Ageton, S. S. (1980). Reconciling race and class differences in self-reported and official estimates of delinquency. *American Sociological Review*, *45*, 95-110.

Elliott, D. S., Huizinga, D., & Ageton, S. S. (1985). *Explaining delinquency and drug use*. Beverly Hills, CA: Sage.

Elliott, R., & Tighe, T. (1968). Breaking the cigarette habit: Effects of a technique involving threatened loss of money. *Psychological Record*, *18*, 503-513.

Eyberg, S. M., & Johnson, S. M. (1974). Multiple assessment of behavior modification with families: Effects of contingency contracting and order of treated problems. *Journal of Consulting and Clinical Psychology*, *42*, 594-606.

Firestone, P., Kelly, M. J., & Fike, S. (1980). Are fathers necessary in parent training groups? *Journal of Clinical Child Psychology*, *9*, 44-47.

Fleishman, M. (1981). A replication of Patterson's "Intervention for boys with conduct problems." *Journal of Consulting and Clinical Psychology*, *49*(3), 342-351.

Fleischman, M. J. (1971). Using parenting salaries to control attrition and cooperation in therapy. *Behavior Therapy*, *10*, 111-116.

Fleischman, M. J. (1979). Training and evaluation of aggressive children. NIMH Proposal. Eugene, OR: Oregon Social Learning Center.

Fleischman, M. J., & Szykula, S. A. (1980). A community setting replication of a social learning treatment for aggressive children. Helena, MT: Family Research Associates, Helena Family Teaching Center (manuscript).

Glogower, R., & Sloop, E. W. (1976). Two strategies of group training of parents as effective behavior modifiers. *Behavior Therapy*, *7*, 177-184.

Gold, J. (1981). Parent and child training model. Seattle, WA: School of Social Work, University of Washington, unpublished doctoral dissertation.

Gordon, T. (1970). *Parent effectiveness training*. New York: Wyden Books.

Griest, D. L., & Wells, K. C. (1983). Behavioral family therapy with conduct disorders in children. *Behavior Therapy*, *14*, 37-53.

Hawkins, J. D., & Salisbury, B. (1983). Delinquency prevention programs for minorities of color. *Social Work Research and Abstracts*, *19*(4), 5-12.

Hawkins, J. D., & Weis, J. G. (1985). The social development model: An integrated approach to delinquency prevention. *Journal of Primary Prevention*, *6*(2), 73-97.

Hawkins, R. P., Peterson, R. F., Schweid, E., & Bijou, S. (1966). Behavior therapy in the home, amelioration of problem parent/child relations with the parent in the therapist's role. *Journal of Experimental Child Psychology*, *4*, 99-107.

Herrnstein, R. J. (1977). The evolution of behaviorism. *American Psychologist*, *32*(8), 593-603.

Hirschi, T. (1969). *Causes of delinquency*. Berkeley, CA: University of California Press.

Humphreys, L., Forehand, R., McMahon, R., & Roberts, M. (1978). Parent behavioral training to modify child noncompliance: Effects on untreated siblings. *Journal of Behavior Therapy and Experimental Psychiatry*, *9*, 235-238.

Janiak, B. P. (1975). An evaluation of the effectiveness of parent training programs in changing parent behavior. Unpublished doctoral dissertation, Utah State University.

Jessor, R., & Jessor, S. L. (1977). *Problem behavior and psychosocial developments: A longitudinal study of youth*. New York: Academic Press.

Johnson, S. M., & Christensen, A. (1975). Multiple criteria follow-up of behavior modification with families. *Journal of Abnormal Child Psychology*, *3*, 135-154.

Karoly, P., & Rosenthal, M. (1977). Training parents in behavior modification: Effects on perceptions of family interaction and deviant child behavior. *Behavior Therapy*, *8*, 406-410.

Klein, N. C., Alexander, J. F., & Parsons, B. V. (1977). Impact of family systems intervention on recidivism and sibling delinquency: A model of primary prevention and program evaluation. *Journal of Consulting and Clinical Psychology*, *45*(3), 469-474.

Lavigueur, H. (1976). The use of siblings as an adjunct to the behavioral treatment of children in the home with parents as therapists. *Behavior Therapy*, *7*, 602-613.

Loeber, R., & Stouthamer-Loeber, M. (1985). Models and metaanalyses of the relationship between family variables and juvenile conduct problems and delinquency. In N. Morris & M. Tonry (Eds.), *Crime and justice: An annual review of research*, Vol. 7. Chicago: University of Chicago Press.

Martin, B. (1977). Brief family therapy intervention: Effectiveness and the importance of including the father. *Journal of Consulting and Clinical Psychology*, *45*(6), 1001-1010.

McCord, J. (1978). A thirty-year follow-up of treatment effects. *Am Psych*, *33*, 284-289.

McMahon, R. J., & Forehand, R. (1978). Nonprescription behavior therapy: Effectiveness of a brochure in teaching mothers to correct their children's inappropriate mealtime behaviors. *Behavior Therapy*, *9*, 814-820.

McMahon, R. J., Forehand, R., & Griest, D. L. (1981). Effects of knowledge of social learning principles on enhancing treatment outcome and generalization in a parent training program. *Journal of Consulting and Clinical Psychology*, *49*, 526-532.

Miles, J. M. H. (1974). A comparative analysis of the effectiveness of verbal reinforcement group counseling and parent effectiveness training on certain behavioral aspects of potential dropout. Unpublished doctoral dissertation, Auburn University.

Moore, D., Chamberlain, P., & Muka, L. (1979). Children at risk for delinquency: A follow-up comparison of aggressive children and children who steal. *Journal of Abnormal Child Psychology*, 7(3), 345-355.

O'Dell, S. L. (1974). Training parents in behavior modification: A review. *Psychological Bulletin*, *81*, 418-433.

O'Dell, S. L., Flynn, J., & Benlolo, L. (1977). A comparison of parent training techniques in child behavior modification. *Journal of Behavior Therapy and Experimental Psychiatry*, *8*, 261-268.

O'Dell, S. C., Mahoney, N. D., Horton, W., & Turner, P. E. (1979). Media assisted parent training: Alternate models. *Behavior Therapy*, *10*, 103-110.

O'Dell, S. L., Drug, W. W., Patterson, J. N., & Fastman, W. (1980). An assessment of methods for training parents in the use of time-out. *Journal of Behavior Therapy and Experimental Psychiatry*, *11*, 21-25.

Oei, T. P., & Jackson, P. R. (1980). Long-term effects of group and individual social skills training with alcoholics. *Addictive Behaviors*, *5*, 129-136.

Parsons, B. V., & Alexander, J. F. (1973). Short-term family intervention: A therapy outcome study. *Journal of Consulting and Clinical Psychology*, *41*, 195-201.

Patterson, G. R. (1974a). Retraining of aggressive boys by the parents: Review of recent literature and follow-up evaluation. *Canadian Psychiatric Association Journal*, *19*, 142-158.

Patterson, G. R. (1974b). Interventions for boys with conduct problems: Multiple

settings, treatment, and criteria. *Journal of Consulting and Clinical Psychology, 42*, 471-481.
Patterson, G. R. (1975). *Families*. Champaign, IL: Research Press.
Patterson, G. R. (1979). Social learning techniques for parents of difficult children. In S. Prestwich, *Families today: Strengthening the family*. DHEW Publication Number (ADM) 79-896, pp. 879-896.
Patterson, G. R. (1982). *Coercive family process*. Eugene, OR: Castalia Press.
Patterson, G. R., Chamberlain, P., & Reid, J. B. (1982). A comparative evaluation of a parent training program. *Behavior Therapy, 13*, 638-650.
Patterson, G. R., & Fleischman, M. J. (1979). Maintenance of treatment effects: Some considerations concerning family systems and follow-up data. *Behavior Therapy, 10*, 168-185.
Patterson, G. R., & Gullian, M. E. (1971). *Living with children*. Champaign, IL: Research Press.
Patterson, G. R., Littman, R. A., & Bricker, W. (1967a). Assertive behavior in children: A step toward a theory of aggression. *Monographs of the Society of Research in Child Development, 32*(5) (Serial No. 113).
Patterson, G. R., McNeal, S., Hawkins, N., & Phelps, R. (1967b). Reprogramming the social environment. *Journal of Child Psychology and Psychiatry, 8*, 181-195.
Patterson, G. R., & Reid, J. B. (1973). Intervention for families of aggressive boys: A replication study. *Behavior Research and Therapy, 11*, 383-394.
Patterson, G. R., & Reid, J. B. (1970). Reciprocity and coercion: Two facets of social systems. In C. Neuringer & J. Michael (Eds.), *Behavior modification in clinical psychology*. New York: Appleton-Century-Crofts.
Patterson, G. R., Reid, J. B., Jones, R. R., & Conger, R. E. (1975). A social learning approach to family intervention. Vol. I. *Families with aggressive children*. Eugene, OR: Castalia Press.
Patterson, G. R., & Stouthamer-Loeber, M. (1984). The correlation of family management practices and delinquency. *Child Development, 55*, 1299-1307.
Pinkston, E. M., & Herbert-Jackson, E. W. (1975). Modification of irrelevant and bizarre verbal behavior using parents as the therapists. *Social Service Review, 49*(1), 46-63.
Powers, E., & Witmer, H. (1951). *An experiment in the prevention of delinquency: The Cambridge-Somerville Youth Study*. New York: Columbia University.
Reid, J. B., & Patterson, G. R. (1976). The modification of aggression and stealing behaviors of boys in the home setting. In E. Ribes & A. Bandura (Eds.), *Analysis of delinquency and aggression*. Hillsdale, NJ: Erlbaum Associates.
Reid, J. B., Hinojosa-Rivero, G., & Loeber, R. (1980). *A social learning approach to the outpatient treatment of children who steal*. Eugene, OR: Oregon Social Learning Center.
Reisman, F. (1965). The "helper" therapy principle. *Social Work, 10*, 27-32.
Rimm, D. C., & Masters, J. C. (1978). *Behavior therapy*. New York: Academic Press.

Roberts, M. W., McMahon, R. J., Forehand, R., & Humphreys, L. (1978). The effect of parental instruction-giving on child compliance. *Behavior Therapy*, *9*, 793-798.

Robin, A. L. (1981). A controlled evaluation of problem-solving communication training with parent-adolescent conflict. *Behavior Therapy*, *12*(5), 593-609.

Robin, A. L., Kent, R., O'Leary, K. D., Foster, S., & Prinz, R. (1977). An approach to teaching parents and adolescents problem-solving communications skills: A preliminary report. *Behavior Therapy*, *8*, 639-643.

Rose, S. D. (1974). Training parents in groups as behavior modifiers of their mentally retarded children. *Journal of Behavior Therapy and Experimental Psychiatry*, *5*, 135-140.

Sanders, M. R., & Glynn, T. (1981). Training parents in behavioral self-management: An analysis of generalization and maintenance. *Journal of Applied Behavior Analysis*, *14*(3), 223-237.

Shapiro, R. (1974). Therapist attitudes and premature termination in family and individual therapy. *Journal of Nervous and Mental Disorders*, *159*, 101-107.

Shaver, J. P., & Nuhn, D. (1971). The effectiveness of tutoring underachievers in reading and writing. *Journal of Educational Research*, *65*, 107-112.

Strain, P. S., Steele, P., Ellis, T., & Tinar, M. (1982). Long-term effects of oppositional child treatment with mothers as therapists and therapist trainers. *Journal of Applied Behavior Analysis*, *15*, 163-169.

Taplin, P. S., & Reid, J. B. (1977). Changes in parent consequation as a function of family intervention. *Journal of Clinical and Consulting Psychology*, *4*, 973-981.

Tighe, T. J., & Elliott, R. A. (1968). A technique for controlling behavior in natural life settings. *Journal of Applied Behavior Analysis*, *1*, 263-266.

Trovato, J., & Bucher, B. (1980). Peer tutoring with or without home-based reinforcement, for reading remediation. *Journal of Applied Behavior Analysis*, *13*(1), 129-141.

Wahler, R. G. (1969a). Oppositional children: A quest for parental reinforcement control. *Journal of Applied Behavior Analysis*, *2*, 159-170.

Wahler, R. G. (1969b). Setting generality: Some specific and general effects of child behavior therapy. *Journal of Applied Behavior Analysis*, *2*, 239-246.

Wahler, R. G. (1980). The insular mother: Her problems in parent-child treatment. *Journal of Applied Behavior Analysis*, *13*(2), 207-219.

Wahler, R. G., Afton, A. D., & Fox, J. J., III (1979). The multiply entrapped parent: Some new problems in parent training. *Education and Treatment of Children*, *2*(4), 279-286.

Weathers, L., & Liberman, R. P. (1975). Contingency contracting with families of delinquent adolescents. *Behavior Therapy*, *6*, 356-366.

Webster-Stratton, C. (1981). Modification of mothers' behaviors and attitudes through a videotape modeling group discussion program. *Behavior Therapy*, *12*(5), 634-642.

Williams, B. F., & Sanders, B. (1974). A comparative study of the relative effectiveness of parent effectiveness training and a program of behavior modification. Department of Psychology, Elon College, North Carolina.

Wilson, J. Q., & Herrnstein, R. N. (1985). *Crime and human nature*. New York: Simon and Schuster.

Wittes, G., & Radin, N. (1971). Two approaches to group work with parents in a compensatory preschool program. *Social Work, 16*, 42-50.

Parents as Intervention Agents for Children with Conduct Problems and Juvenile Offenders

Magda Stouthamer-Loeber
Rolf Loeber

ABSTRACT. Selected research findings on conduct problems and juvenile delinquency that are relevant for practitioners making decisions about the treatment of children with these problems are summarized, with a focus on two decisions: whether to intervene and how to intervene using parents as change agents. The importance of careful assessment, not only of the child's behavior, but also of the parents' strengths and limitations is stressed, along with the importance of flexibility in treatment rather than strict adherence to one theoretical model. Important considerations in assessment and treatment are discussed.

The focus of this article has been restricted to interventions with children with conduct problems using parents as change agents for two reasons. First, teaching parents different child rearing techniques in order to change their children's behavior is one of the most widely used intervention strategies, especially for younger children. Second, in an area where successful treatment is not always common, this intervention strategy has met with reasonable success (Berkowitz & Graziano, 1972; Johnson & Katz, 1974; Moreland, Schwebel, Beck, & Wells, 1982), and with more success than many other treatment modes (Kazdin, 1984; Loeber, 1984).

Magda Stouthamer-Loeber and Rolf Loeber are affiliated with the Western Psychiatric Institute and Clinic, University of Pittsburgh School of Medicine, 3811 O'Hara Street, Pittsburgh, PA 15213.

PRE-INTERVENTION ASSESSMENT

The decision to try to reduce a child's problem behavior is influenced by a number of factors, such as the current seriousness of the child's behavior, the expected course of development, the expected chance of success, and parental concern about the behavior. How to intervene is another matter, which requires taking into consideration additional factors such as the child's age, parents' willingness to make changes, and their ability to do so.

What are serious conduct problems? The answer to this question depends to some extent on the child's age. A six-month-old baby who kicks and screams to make his or her displeasure known, for example, will not be called conduct disordered. The behavior is normal for this age; the child has not yet learned alternative and more adaptive ways to express feelings or to control the environment. However, if a six-year-old consistently shows this behavior, there is reason for concern. Patterson (1982) calls this arrested socialization. In other words, some behaviors, like screaming, kicking, biting, grabbing, and fighting, which are relatively normal at an early age are in most children gradually replaced by more socially acceptable behaviors. Those children who have not learned to make that switch, may be in need of treatment.

Conduct problems do not only consist of immature behaviors. As children grow older, the repertoire of possible conduct problems widens. This expansion is thought to follow a somewhat predictable, developmental pattern (Edelbrock & Loeber, 1985). There are, as it were, age-appropriate conduct problems, which have a higher chance of occurring if other problem behaviors have preceded them. Because of this predictability, seriousness of a problem behavior almost always partly refers to its prognosis in addition to its present nuisance value.

Several criteria can be used to assess the seriousness of conduct behaviors: density, variety, time of onset, and number of different settings in which the behaviors occur (Loeber, 1982). Density refers to the frequency of conduct behaviors. Obviously, the more a child lies, fights, or steals, the more one should be concerned that this is not a passing phase. The number of different kinds of problem behaviors that a child engages in is also related to future outcome. For instance, children who fight *and* steal are expected to have a worse prognosis than those who only fight or only steal.

If the behavior has generalized to more than one setting, e.g., home *and* school, it is considered to be less under control of specific environmental stimuli, and therefore less tractable. A very important indicator of seriousness is early onset. Children who, relative to their peers, engage early in serious antisocial behaviors are more likely to continue than those who start much later. This is particularly the case for delinquency where a large number of studies have shown that a chronic delinquent career is associated with an early start (see Loeber, 1982).

The more serious the child behavior is according to the above criteria, the more the child is in need of treatment. However, practitioners know all too well that those most in need of treatment are often those that are most difficult to help. The environmental handicaps that seem to maintain the behavior and the long-standing ingrainedness of the behaviors themselves may prove to be hard to overcome. The younger children are, the more successful one might be in deflecting them from a path of increasingly more practiced problem behaviors. Also parents of younger children might be less set in dealing with their children in ways that may not be optimal. Parents also still have potentially more control over younger than older children.

Not all child problem behaviors affect the parents in the same way (Loeber & Schmaling, 1985). Overt or confrontive behaviors, such as fighting, bullying, and temper tantrums may give rise to immediate irritations, because they affect the parents directly. These are behaviors that cannot be ignored very easily. Parents may find the behavior irritating enough to seek treatment. On the other hand, covert, or concealing behaviors, such as lying, stealing, truancy and drug use, are by their nature not immediately obvious. Parents may initially try to ignore the behaviors and give the child the benefit of the doubt. Even when they find out what the child has been up to, parents may be at a loss as to how they should react to a behavior that most likely took place a while ago. Often parents seek help only when pressed to do so by the school or other official agencies.

Many volumes have been written on the assessment of child behavior (Brodsky & Smitherman, 1983; Mash & Terdal, 1981; Ollendick & Hersen, 1984; Orvaschel, Sholomskas, & Weissman, 1980), and several widely used scales are available, such as the *Child Behavior Check List* (Achenbach & Edelbrock, 1981), *Teacher Report Form* (Edelbrock & Achenbach, 1984), *Self-reported Delinquency Questionnaire* (Elliot, Huizinga, & Ageton, 1985), *Conners' Parents Questionnaire* (Conners, 1970), and the *Behavior Problem Checklist* (Quay & Peterson, 1967). However, these behavior rating scales need to be supplemented by questions about onset of behavior and number of different settings in which the behavior occurs. Also, most scales measure aggressive behaviors relatively well but are not very strong on the measurement of covert or concealing behaviors.

Besides assessing the *children's behavior* carefully before deciding on treatment, the *parents' behavior and attitudes* need to be scrutinized with equal care, especially if one is contemplating using the parents as change agents. Failure to do so may lead to less than optimal treatment outcome (Griest & Wells, 1983). It is necessary to establish the parents' actual and potential strengths in child rearing, and their limitations as they may be related to the child's problem behaviors.

Before the parents can be expected to make the effort to try to change the child, they need to realize the seriousness of the child's behavior. They may not be aware of what the child is heading for, their standards may be different, or they may feel that they have no control over the child's development. Therefore, parents need to *want* the child's behavior to be changed and need to be given the feeling that they *can* do it.

The cooperation of parents can easily be destroyed if they get the feeling during the assessment phase or in the later treatment that they are the ones to blame for the child's predicament. It is well to remember that most parents do not consciously set out to create a problem child. They would certainly prefer to have an easy child. Although our orientation may lead us to believe that parenting skill deficits lead to child problem behaviors, this unidirectional model is not sufficient (Bell, 1968). One should keep in mind that children come into this world equipped with different temperaments, and some children are harder to handle than others (Cameron, 1978). It is quite likely that some of the children that practitioners see professionally might sorely try even their child rearing techniques if they had to live with them on a daily basis.

The measurement of parent behaviors is not as well developed as that of child behaviors. Each of the survey studies in our literature review that will be discussed below used its own questions, and no generally accepted assessment package for measuring parent behavior has emerged. To be sure, there is a myriad of scales that measure some aspect(s) of parental functioning, such as the *Children's Reports of Parental Behavior* (Schaefer, 1965), *The Family Environment Scale* (Moos, 1975), and the *Dyadic Adjustment Scale* (Spanier, 1976), to mention just a few. At present, we are working on a more comprehensive set of measures for parent behaviors in order to try and fill this gap, but at the moment, practitioners have to rely to some extent on their own ingenuity to assess parents.

Parental Behaviors and Conditions Related to Child Conduct Problems

In this section we will discuss the empirical evidence that exists for a connection between parent behaviors and circumstances, and child problem behavior. We will draw mainly from two extensive reviews of the empirical literature (Loeber & Dishion, 1983; Loeber & Stouthamer-Loeber, in press) and will summarize a part of their findings. The studies reviewed in the two papers mainly concern delinquency (official or self-reported), and therefore do not pertain to preschoolers. Also, many studies have included only boys, so the evidence for girls is much scarcer.

Obviously, reviews of the literature are never complete. Material is presented through the filter of the reviewer as well as the filter of the original researcher. These filters reflect partly the philosophy of our time and partly individual idiosyncrasies (Scarr, 1985). Our choice of variables was determined by the following. As a practitioner, one is interested in pinpointing circumstances that caused, or better still, maintain the undesirable behavior. Such information is maximally useful if the circumstance in question is potentially amenable to change. Therefore, variables such as socioeconomic status or race, may be related to certain conduct problems but cannot form the target for intervention, and have been left out of the review.

In order to structure the mass of data, we have used four models of family influence: Neglect, Conflict, Deviant Parental Values, and Family Disruption. These four models represent different avenues by which parents are thought to influence their children's problem behavior. The first two models concern socialization practices by parents directed at their children, whereas the last two models concern background variables, i.e., parent behaviors or circumstances that are not necessarily aimed at children but might influence them nevertheless. The models should not be seen as mutually exclusive. On the contrary, often two or more of them co-occur or evolve from each other over time. Before we present the summary of the literature reviews, we will discuss the four models.

Neglect

Parents need to spend a certain amount of time with children as a necessary, although not sufficient, condition for successful child rearing. The parents' involvement with children can take several forms, such as doing activities or games together, going on outings, or just spending time talking to each other. Being actively involved with the child gives parents an opportunity to teach the child socially acceptable skills and creates a possibility for mutual attachment and appreciation.

Moreover, parents who do not spent sufficient time with their children are not in a position to supervise their children. When children are small, supervision takes place by personally being present. As they grow older, supervision will start to include being informed as to where the child is, with whom, and what his/her activities are when away from home. Lack of supervision makes it impossible to guide children's activities by advice, reinforcement, punishment, and the setting of rules. However, just being in the child's proximity does not necessarily make a parent pay attention or discuss what the child is planning to do when away from home. Supervision is rather more active, and also presupposes a set of standards that parents want to adhere to. These standards range from "I don't want my child to swallow bleach" to "I don't want my child to be out after dark." When there are very few or no rules or standards, supervision becomes an empty concept.

Conflict

In most families, parents and children get into conflict at times. However, in some families conflict is a way of life, because the child is temperamentally exceptionally difficult, and/or because of a lack of parenting skill. Parents may not have learned effective means of making their children behave appropriately. Problems may be dealt with in a confrontive, verbally aggressive, and possibly even a physically aggressive manner because parents approach all their problems like that. Their discipline techniques may be inadequate, too intermittently used, or inconsistent in the face of opposition.

Some children have learned to escalate their problem behaviors in the face of parental efforts to control them. These counter control moves may cause parents to back off, and even to be afraid of the child. The immediate cost of imposing control has become too high. In these cases there may not be open conflict because the parents have basically given up on their parenting role. Regardless of the source(s) of the conflict, continuing problems pitch the battling parties against each other and cause them to perceive each other as enemies. Therefore, conflict may be accompanied or followed by rejection of each other. Direct conflict has rarely been measured in the survey studies discussed below. However, discipline and rejection, the other aspects of this model have frequently been measured.

Deviant Parental Values

Deviant or antisocial parental values can have their effect on children in two ways. First, parents by their own behavior may *model* deviant behavior which their children may adopt. Second, parents with a different value system might *not punish or discourage* deviant behaviors, and therefore deprive their children of the consequences that most children who engage in such behaviors experience. For instance, parents with deviant values might protect their children from the police, or not pay attention when goods of uncertain provenance are brought into the house. Parents might even actively teach children to be aggressive or "tough," with the idea that real boys should be able to stand up for themselves.

In contrast to the first two models where parents and children are either not in contact or are in conflict, this model assumes a degree of concordance between parents and children, at least about some aspects of the child's behavior. This is not the case for another set of parental values, such as expectations that are too high for their children in terms of age or abilities. Unrealistic expectations may lead parents to reject the child and can be a source of continuous conflict.

Family Disruption

Neglect and conflict may occur when family members are under the stress of unusual events, such as serious illness, marital conflict or marital break-up. Under such circumstances, parents may have less time or inclination to concern themselves with their children. In addition the stress under which they live may have made them irritable so that interactions may easily lead to conflict with their children. Once the stressors have been removed, parents may revert to more favorable child rearing practices. However, for some families, disruptions are a chronic pattern.

Important Studies on Family and Delinquency

In the following section, where we will summarize the literature on the relationship of family variables and delinquency and conduct problems, two kinds of evidence will be presented. Some studies address *concurrent* relationships between the parent variables and child behavior, whereas other studies present *predictive* data. In the latter case parent variables are used to predict child behavior at a later date. A further distinction can be made with regard to the subjects used. Some studies contrast official delinquents with nondelinquents, and other studies sample from the whole range of children. These latter studies usually try to explain youngsters' self-reported delinquency rather than official delinquency. If parent behaviors are related to child conduct problems, it is expected that this relationship will emerge more strongly in studies with official, rather than self-reported delinquency, since the officially delinquent children are most likely more extreme in terms of problem behavior. Also, studies with contrasting groups rather than normal samples will yield stronger differences in parent behaviors.

Different studies use different statistics which make it difficult to compare the outcomes. In the review articles a new measure, Relative Improvement Over Chance (RIOC) was used which made it possible to compare the results among studies. RIOC is expressed as a percentage of improvement over chance by using one variable to predict another (Loeber & Dishion, 1983). For the sake of simplicity, only studies which could be converted to RIOC will be summarized here.

Table 1 shows a summary of 45 studies reviewed in Loeber and Stouthamer-Loeber (in press). In general, the socialization vari-

Table 1

Summary of Familial Variables Associated with Child Conduct Problems and Delinquency

Variable	Concurrent: Comparison median RIOC	Concurrent: Normal median RIOC	Predictive: Normal median RIOC
Parent-child involvement	61.5	-	31.0
Child-parent involvement	49.3	18.3	-
Supervision	66.3	14.6	36.4
Discipline	73.5	11.6	17.6
Parental rejection	62.6	24.0	35.8
Child rejection of parent	56.3	22.9	-
Parental criminality, deviant values, or aggressiveness	34.5	23.6	22.5
Marital relations	29.1	23.3	28.0
Parental absence	27.7	12.5	12.2
Parental health	28.0	10.6	16.5
Composite family factors	-	-	57.5

Note. Adapted from "Family factors as correlates and predictors of juvenile conduct problems and delinquency" by R. Loeber and M. Stouthamer-Loeber, 1986. In N. Morris and M. Tonry (Eds.) Crime and justice: An annual review of research. (Vol. 7). Chicago: University of Chicago Press.

ables embodied in the first two models and reflecting the quality and quantity of parent-child interaction were more strongly related to child conduct problems and delinquency than the background variables of the last two models. This is especially the case in concurrent studies using comparison samples of official delinquents and nondelinquents. The RIOCs for socialization variables such as involvement, supervision, discipline, and rejection were roughly twice as large as those for background variables, such as parental deviant values, marital relations, parental absence, and parental health, ranging from 49.3 to 73.5% and 27.7 to 34.5%, respectively.

As expected, concurrent studies that used contrasting comparison groups of official delinquents and nondelinquents showed stronger relationships than studies using normal samples with self-reported delinquency as dependent variable. The ranking of the median RIOCs was somewhat different. The highest variables were parental rejection (24.0%), parental criminality (23.6%), and marital discord (23.3%).

Turning to predictive studies, most of them consisted of relatively normal samples rather than contrasting groups. With the exception of discipline, the RIOC ranking of the variables was very similar to the ranking using the concurrent comparison studies. In psychology it is usual to find that relationships decrease in strength as the time interval increases between the measurement of two variables, because of the effect of other variables that have appeared in the interval. However, this was not the case for a number of parenting variables. Lack of supervision in particular, but to a lesser extent also inappropriate discipline, parental rejection, marital problems, and parental ill health, were all more strongly related to *later* than to *concurrent* child conduct problems and delinquency. This probably reflects the cumulative influence of these variables when they are in effect over a long period of time.

As was mentioned, the four models do not operate in a mutually exclusive way. Often several parenting skills or circumstances are less than optimal, and deficits in parenting may coincide. A number of researchers have documented medium-level intercorrelations between various parenting deficits (Hirschi, 1969; Kagan & Moss, 1962; McCord, 1982; Patterson & Stouthamer-Loeber, 1984).

If parenting deficits coincide, do they have a cumulative effect on the child's behavior? Predictive studies using a composite measure of family factors, combining from two to seven variables, suggest that this is the case. Composite family factors yielded the highest median RIOC (57.5%) for the predictive studies. The combined effect of family factors is well illustrated in the earlier review (Loeber & Dishion, 1983), where composite measures of family factors were the strongest predictors of delinquency, surpassing even child problem behavior.

Cumulative effects often occur because different aspects of models evolve over time. For instance, parents' poor supervision may lead to serious child problem behavior which may be the cause for continuous conflict. Or families, exhausted by chronic fighting may turn to rejection and neglect.

Different levels of seriousness of child behavior are related to different levels of seriousness of parental handicap. Studies using self-reported delinquency as a criterion had RIOCs that were on average half as large as those that used official delinquency. Even stronger evidence for this position comes from a study by Patterson and Stouthamer-Loeber (1984) who found that 21% of the nondelinquents were poorly monitored by their parent(s) compared to 50% and 73% for the one-to-two time offenders and multiple offenders, respectively. In the case of self-reported delinquency, the percentages of poorly supervised children were 10%, 30%, and 76%, respectively.

Earlier, we made a distinction between overt, or confrontive conduct problems and covert, or concealing ones. In terms of accompanying parent behavior, this distinction seems to have some validity. The review of the literature revealed some support for differential parenting deficits associated with each. Covert conduct problems seemed to be associated more with parental neglect and lack of open conflict. Overt conduct problems were found more in families with chronic conflict among all family members, and particularly with the child.

It should be kept in mind that correlational studies, even longitudinal ones, only present information on the relationship between conduct problems and other variables. They do not provide hard evidence about the causal relationship between the two. This is not to say that such information is useless. It presents practitioners with raw material for working hypotheses about what might change a child's behavior.

TREATING CONDUCT DISORDERS USING FAMILY INTERVENTION

Considering the large variety of parenting deficits that may occur singly or in combination, the necessity of a thorough assessment and a flexible treatment approach should stand out very clearly. We will discuss the implications for treatment of deficits in parenting in each of the four models. Many of the actual techniques are described in a number of parent training manuals (Fleischman, Horne, & Arthur, 1983; Forehand & McMahon, 1981; Patterson, 1977; Patterson, Reid, Jones, & Conger, 1975; Reid, 1978).

Parental Supervision and Involvement to Overcome Neglect

Different kinds of supervision are necessary for children at different ages. For very young children supervision may mean making sure that the child really finishes his/her plate when told to do so, being aware of what the child watches on TV, or glancing out of the kitchen window every few minutes when the child is playing in the backyard. With young children, it is largely a matter of being there and paying attention.

Older children spend less and less time in the immediate vicinity of their parents, and supervision takes on a different aspect. Supervision may be expressed in discussing the child's plans for the day, insisting on being informed as to where the child will be, with whom, and what s/he will be doing. It also may mean checking up on the proper adherence to certain rules, such as what time to come home. As was mentioned earlier, a lack of appropriate supervision is often found to accompany covert conduct problems.

Some parents have not learned how to supervise, i.e., what to watch out for. In other cases, supervision is not totally lacking, but the child dodges attempts at supervision. Some children are very skillful at lying about their whereabouts and activities. Other children go even a step further and make the parents feel guilty for even questioning their "good" conduct. Parents who find themselves in this position may need to use supervision that goes beyond verbal inquiries of the child.

Reid, Hinojosa-Rivero and Lorber (1980) used a method of supervision with children who stole that seemed to be quite effective. Instead of listening to ingenious explanations when the child brought home something that the parents had not sen before, parents were instructed to require more positive proof. This proof could consist of a cash receipt for things supposedly bought, a note from the teacher if it had been won at school, a note from somebody's mother if it had been exchanged, etc. This system has several advantages once the ground rules are laid out. First, parents have made the child responsible for the proof, rather than playing the detective themselves. Second, uncertainty is taken away since, if the child cannot provide positive proof, the item will be considered stolen. A similar system can be set up for children who consistently and seriously dodge their parents' attempts to find out where they are and what they are doing, by having them bring home a slip signed by an adult stating where they were. Of course, it is essential to the success of such an intervention that parents have some clear sanctions that are actually imposed when the child is found wanting.

In considering the amount of supervision necessary for a child, it is important to take the child's environment into account. In certain neighborhoods the temptations to deviate may be fewer than, for instance, in an inner city slum. Wilson (1980) found that under the latter circumstances exceedingly strict supervision is necessary to prevent children from getting into problems. This very strict supervision was found to be even more important than a warm and stable home.

Behaviorally oriented psychologists have not paid much attention to the concept of parent-child involvement. However, the concept has played a key role in sociological theories about deviancy (Hirschi, 1969), and has been measured in numerous survey studies. In the review of the literature, lack of involvement between parents and children was strongly related to delinquency and conduct problem behavior in children. It is not always easy to increase involvement, especially if a lack of it is accompanied by conflict and/or rejection.

In young children, the decision to have more involvement can be taken by the parent(s) unilaterally. However, older children might resent this sudden attention, and be suspicious of it. More involvement does not have to mean complicated or costly outings, but any situation which affords the parent and the child time together in a positive, or at least neutral, manner. It can serve as a balance for the less good times, and may help both parents and children to see each other in a less antagonistic light. This will be discussed further under Rejection in the next model.

Parenting Skills for Dealing with Conflict

Improve Communication

One of the mechanisms that may influence the rate of conflict between parents and conduct problem children is the parents' practice of issuing commands at a high rate which are either vague or are immediately contradicted, leaving the child with no good opportunity to comply (Patterson, 1982; Peed, Roberts, & Forehand, 1977). In such cases, part of the treatment will consist of teaching the parents to issue commands only when they really want them executed, and to make the commands clear as to content and time frame. As children grow older, their say in decisions about themselves should increase.

Often problems arise because of the fact that parents and children have different ideas about the extent of the children's part in the decision-making process, or about the process itself. The decision to teach parents and children better negotiating skills and conflict resolution techniques depends on how far the situation has deteriorated. Some conduct problem children so completely terrorize their families that parents are not in a position to negotiate and the children have no need to. In such situations, teaching better negotiating and conflict resolution skills may be postponed and attention given to having the parents regain control over their household, such as advocated by the Toughlove movement (York, York, & Wachtel, 1984). In less extreme cases, the primary goal may well be to reduce the level of conflict. Often, especially when the child is older, this will require family therapy, rather than the training of parents only. With younger children, parents can be taught how to reduce the frequency and length of conflicts by having clear rules and commands, clear consequences which are enforced, and disengagement through the use of time-out when conflict arises.

Improve Discipline

The term discipline has been used for a wide variety of child rearing practices. In some studies the term covers the kind of consequences that parents apply, whereas in other studies discipline refers to the consistency with which parents apply certain measures. In behaviorally oriented treatments for conduct problem children, both aspects receive strong emphasis, and the literature is replete with examples of how to teach parents to pinpoint problem behavior, to use nonphysical punishment, and to be consistent (see e.g., Forehand & McMahon, 1981; Fleischman, Horne, & Arthur, 1983). Nonphysical punishments that are often used are time-out and loss of privileges. This form of intervention is suitable for changing overt conduct problems, such as fighting and disobedience, but, by itself, is less suited for changing covert conduct problems (Loeber, 1984). In order to change covert behavior problems, vigilance and supervision are necessary in order to establish that the undesirable behavior occurred before it can be punished.

Therapists who train parents in better child managing techniques need to make parents aware that their problem child, who has more or less had his or her way for a long time, most likely will not take a change in regime without a fight. Parents need to be prepared for the possibility that the child may get worse instead of better initially, and the parents may need a lot of support to stand up to the temporary escalation.

Decrease Rejection

Parents of problem children may be so preoccupied with trying to straighten out the child's bad behavior, that their whole perception of the child may be colored. As a result, they may miss or disregard the times that the child's behavior is neutral or even good, and think of him or her as all bad. The child may reciprocate these feelings, and both parents and child may find themselves in a spiral where behaviors as well as intentions of the other party are always interpreted as negative. One of the most common complaints that children have about their parents is that they are always down on them and that they can do nothing right in their parents' eyes. This rejection from both sides makes it difficult to focus on the real problems. In order to break this downward movement, parents can be taught to notice the things that are positive about their child, and offer praise when he or she has done something right. Often parents are surprised to find that there are a number of things praiseworthy about their child. This new appreciation, however small, may motivate the parties to work on resolving the actual problems.

Apart from generally trying to notice more positive things about the child, positive attention has also been used as a specific technique to strengthen behaviors that are the opposite of, or incompatible with the problem behavior (Forehand & King, 1977). It has been shown that parents give reinforcement techniques the highest acceptability rating compared to other treatment techniques. Additionally, training parents first in paying attention and using rewards strengthens the effect of more negative consequences, such as time-out when they are added to the treatment plan (Walle, Hobbs, & Caldwell, 1984).

Rejection, especially of older children, may be so complete that the parties may not even want to contemplate the thought that the other person is not totally reprehensible. In those cases, the therapist cannot appeal to the parents' positive feelings towards the child in order to motivate them to work on changing the child's behavior. The only motivation that may be left is self-interest, such as how to be able to live in the same house, how to be bothered less, etc. It may be necessary to first work out with the parents and child some rules for an armistice before any other steps can take place.

Sometimes parental rejection stems from unrealistic expectations of achievement or incomplete understanding of developmental norms. Parents in this category need to be taught what is normal for a child of the abilities and age of their child.

Deviant Parental Values

Unlike the variables discussed thus far, the variables in the next two models do not concern the direct interaction between parents and children, and are therefore more difficult to incorporate into the treatment. When parents come to see a therapist because of their child's problem behavior, they would like to have something done about the *child*. They may concede that if they dealt with the child differently the child's behavior might change. Therefore, the socialization variables of the first two models are good starting points. The variables to be discussed presently focus directly on the parents, and need to be introduced carefully, if they are going to play an important role in the treatment.

As has been mentioned, parents may hold values and show behaviors that are commonly called deviant. Some of the parents may actively advocate these ideas and behaviors. For instance, some parents might encourage their children to bring home stolen goods, or teach them how to pick pockets. Other parents may insist on their children being aggressive, and being good fighters. If not only the parents, but a majority of people in the neighborhood, subscribe to this view, it is difficult to instill alternative values in either the parents or the children. However, most parents still believe in the American Dream. They themselves might not have made it, but they sure would like their children to be successful and respectable.

We don't know of any treatment that is specifically directed at changing the parents' values and deviant behaviors, but in most behaviorally oriented treatments a subtle process of influencing parents' values and behaviors takes place, by showing them alternatives. This is easier to do for aggressive behaviors, where the alternative, such as walking away from a fight, or negotiating a solution, might have some immediate payoff. It is more difficult with covert behaviors such as stealing or not lying, where the alternative, not stealing or lying has no immediate payoff. If a change in attitudes of the parents is one of the important goals of treatment, group sessions with other parents will probably be more successful than individual attention.

Family Disruption

Marital Problems and Single Parent Families

For a number of decades the notion was widely accepted that children from single-parent families were more at risk for conduct problems and delinquency than were children from families with two parents (Ferguson, 1952; Gregory, 1965; Monahan, 1957; Willie, 1967). However, several reviews have suggested that marital discord and home climate were more strongly related to antisocial child behavior than single-parent status (Bane, 1976; Goetting, 1981; Blechman, 1982; Herzog & Sudia, 1973, see also Table 1). Additional evidence comes from a study by Hetherington, Cox, and Cox (1978) who found that children, especially boys, immediately after divorce, showed more behavior problems but that in the course of a few years these behavior problems were substantially reduced. Therefore, parental absence, although certainly not ideal, seems to be less worrisome with regard to the impact on the child's behavior than continuous marital strife.

It is, of course, possible to make the marital problems an additional focus in therapy. However, parents may not want such close scrutiny of their own lives. Although this refusal may make treatment more difficult, there are still some avenues that can be pursued. Stouthamer-Loeber, Schmaling, and Loeber (1984) found in a study of 10- to 16-year-old boys that single mothers as well as unhappily married mothers supervised their children significantly less than happily married mothers. These mothers also had a more negative attitude towards their children. Related findings were reported by Goldstein (1984) who noted that for youths in father absent homes the level of supervision was the crucial factor in the probability of police contacts.

It might, therefore, be helpful to focus on supervision, involvement, and less rejection. Because of the stress these parents may be under, they might find it difficult to have enough time and energy to execute their parenting functions properly. In such cases, it would be useful to explore whether other relatives, neighbors, or organizations might take over some of these functions. This could take the form of the child spending weekends with relatives, dropping in after school at a neighbor's house when there is no parent at home, or being enrolled in an after-school program.

Parental Health

Parental health can be impaired in two major ways: physically and mentally. We know of no studies showing how physical illness affects parenting. However, it is easy to imagine that ill health may have somewhat the same effect as the other family disruptions, i.e., lack of supervision, and lack of involvement. More work has been done on the effects of mental illness on parenting. For instance, depressed mothers have been found to be less consistent in their discipline and more rejecting (Susman, Trickett, Ianotti, Hollenbeck, & Zahn-Waxler, 1985). In another study, depressed mothers were less responsive to their children's dependency needs, and more hostile, dominating, and negative compared to nondepressed mothers (Longfellow, Zelkowitz, & Saunders, 1982). Thus, depressed mothers may exhibit considerable parenting handicaps. If the other parent is not in a position to compensate for the parenting deficits of the spouse, it is necessary to look for outside alternatives, such as were mentioned above.

CONCLUDING COMMENTS

The great variety of possible interventions that have briefly been touched upon in the preceding section may be somewhat overwhelming. However, as has been stressed before, the choice is not random, and depends to a large extent on a thorough pre-intervention assessment of both child and parents, and a continued sensitivity to new problems and information as the treatment unfolds. It should be clear that it is unprofitable to stick to one particular training plan to fit all families. Therefore, although parent training manuals are very useful and generally incorporate the "best bets" in terms of hypotheses about behavior change, practitioners need to maintain an open mind in regard both to reasons why behavior change is not proceeding according to plan, and to what else can be done. This tailoring of treatment, taking into account children's particular behaviors as well as parents' strengths and weaknesses in a number of areas, will increase the likelihood of a favorable outcome.

REFERENCES

Achenbach, T. M., & Edelbrock, C. S. (1981). Behavioral problems and competencies reported by parents of normal and disturbed children aged four through sixteen. *Monograph of the Society for Research in Child Development*, *46*, 1-82.

Bane, M. J. (1976). Marital disruption and the lives of children. *Journal of Social Issues*, *32*, 103-117.

Bell, R. Q. (1968). A reinterpretation of the direction of effects in studies of socialization. *Psychological Review*, *75*, 81-95.

Berkowitz, B. P., & Graziano, A. M. (1972). Training parents as behavior therapists: A review. *Behavior Research and Therapy*, *10*, 297-317.

Blechman, E. (1982). Are children with one parent at psychological risk? A methodological review. *Journal of Marriage and the Family*, *44*, 179-195.

Brodsky, S. L., & Smitherman, H. O'N. (Eds.).(1983). *Handbook of scales for research in crime and delinquency*. New Yoık: Plenum.

Cameron, J. R. (1978). Parental treatment, children's temperament, and the risk of childhood behavioral problems: 2. Initial temperament, parental attitudes and the incidence and form of behavioral problems. *American Journal of Orthopsychiatry*, *48*, 140-147.

Conners, C. K. (1970). Symptom patterns in hyperkinetic, neurotic, and normal children. *Child Development*, *41*, 667-682.

Edelbrock, C., & Achenbach, T. M. (1984). The teacher version of the Child Behavior Profile: I. Boys aged 6-11. *Journal of Consulting and Clinical Psychology*, *52*, 207-217.

Edelbrock, C., & Loeber, R. (1985). *The development of antisocial behavior in childhood and adolescence*. Unpublished manuscript, University of Massachusetts Medical School, Worcester, MA.

Elliott, D. S., Huizinga, D., & Ageton, S. S. (1985). *Explaining delinquency and drug use*. Beverly Hills: Sage.

Ferguson, T. (1952). *The gang delinquent in his social setting*. London: Oxford University Press.

Fleischman, M. J., Horne, A. M., & Arthur, J. L. (1983). *Troubled families: A treatment program*. Champaign, IL: Research Press.

Forehand, R., & King, H. E. (1977). Noncompliant children. *Behavior Modification*, *1*, 93-108.

Forehand, R., & McMahon, R. J. (1981). *Helping the noncompliant child: A clinician's guide to parent training*. New York; Guilford.

Goetting, A. (1981). Divorce outcome research. *Journal of Family Issues*, *2*, 350-378.

Goldstein, H. S. (1984). Parental composition, supervision, and conduct problems in youths 12 to 17 years old. *Journal of the American Academy of Child Psychiatry*, *23*, 679-684.

Gregory, J. (1965). Anterospective data following childhood loss of a parent. I. Delinquency and high school dropout. *Archives of General Psychiatry*, *13*, 99-109.

Griest, D. L., & Wells, K. C. (1983). Behavioral family therapy with conduct disorders in children. *Behavior Therapy*, *14*, 37-53.

Herzog, E., & Sudia, C. E. (1973). Children in fatherless families. In B. M. Caldwell and H. N. Ricciuti (Eds.), *Review of child development* (vol. 3). Chicago, IL: University of Chicago Press.

Hetherington, E. M., Cox, M., & Cox, R. (1977). The aftermath of divorce. In J.

H. Stevens, Jr., and M. Matthews (Eds.), *Mother/child, father/child relations*. Washington, DC: National Association for the Education of Young Children.

Hirschi, T. (1969). *Causes of delinquency*. Berkeley: University of California Press.

Johnson, S. A., & Katz, R. C. (1973). Using parents as change agents for their children: A review. *Journal of Child Psychology and Psychiatry*, *4*, 181-200.

Kagan, J., & Moss, H. A. (1962). *Birth to maturity*. New York: Wiley.

Kazdin, A. E. (1984). Treatment of conduct disorders. In J. B. W. Williams & R. L. Spitzer (Eds.), *Psychotherapy research: Where are we going*? New York: Guilford, 3-27.

Loeber, R. (1982). The stability of antisocial and delinquent child behavior: A review. *Child Development*, *53*, 1431-1446.

Loeber, R. (1984). *Experimental studies to reduce antisocial and delinquent child behavior: Implications for future programs and optimal times for intervention*. Paper presented at the ADAMHA/OJJDP Conference on Juvenile Offenders with Serious Drug, Alcohol and Mental Health Problems. Bethesda, MD.

Loeber, R., & Dishion, T. J. (1983). Early predictors of male delinquency: A review. *Psychological Bulletin*, *94*, 68-99.

Loeber, R., & Schmaling, K. B. (1985). The utility of differentiating between mixed and pure forms of antisocial child behavior. *Journal of Abnormal Child Behavior*, *13*, 315-336.

Loeber, R., & Stouthamer-Loeber, M. (in press). Models and meta analyses of the relationship between family variables and juvenile conduct problems and delinquency. In N. Morris and M. Tonry (Eds.), *Crime and justice: An annual review of research* (vol. 7). Chicago, IL: University of Chicago Press.

Longfellow, C., Zelkowitz, P., & Saunders, E. (1982). The quality of mother-child relationships. In D. Belle (Ed.), *Lives in stress*. Beverly Hills, CA: Sage.

McCord, J. (1982). A longitudinal study of the link between broken homes and criminality. In J. Gunn & D. Farrington (Eds.), *Abnormal offenders, delinquency, and the criminal justice system*. London: Wiley.

Mash, E. J., & Terdal, L. G. (Eds.).(1981). *Behavioral assessment of childhood disorders*. New York: Guilford.

Monahan, T. P. (1957). Family status and delinquency. *Social Forces*, *35*, 250-258.

Moos, R. H. (1975). *Evaluating correctional and community settings*. New York: Wiley.

Moreland, S. R., Schwebel, A. I., Beck, S., & Wells, R. T. (1982). Parents as therapists: A review of the behavior therapy parent training literature 1975 to 1981. *Behavior Modification*, *6*, 250-276.

Ollendick, T. H., & Hersen, M. (Eds.).(1984). *Child behavior assessment. Principles and procedures*. New York: Pergamon Press.

Orvaschel, H., Sholomskas, D., & Weissman, M. M. (1980). *NIMH, Series AN No 1. The assessment of psychopathology and the behavioral problems in children: A review of scales suitable for epidemiological and clinical research*

(1967-1979). DHHS Publication No (ADM) 80-1037. Superintendent of Documents, U.S. Government Printing Office, Washington, DC.
Patterson, G. R. (1982). *A social learning approach, Vol. 3; Coercive family process*. Eugene, OR: Castalia Publishing Company.
Patterson, G. R. (1977). *Living with children* (rev. ed.). Champaign, IL: Research Press.
Patterson, G. R., Reid, J. B., Jones, R. R., & Conger, R. E. (1975). *A social learning approach to family intervention, volume I, families with aggressive children*. Eugene, OR: Castalia Press.
Patterson, G. R., & Stouthamer-Loeber, M. (1984). The correlation of family management practices and delinquency. *Child Development*, *55*, 1299-1307.
Peed, S., Roberts, M., & Forehand, R. (1977). Evaluation of the effectiveness of a standardized parent training program in altering the interaction of mothers and their noncompliant children. *Behavior Modification*, *1*, 323-350.
Quay, H. C., & Peterson, D. R. (1967). *Manual for the Behavior Problem Checklist*. Champaign, IL: University of Illinois, Child Research Center.
Reid, J. B. (Ed.).(1978). *A social learning approach to family intervention, vol. 2: Observation in home settings*. Eugene, OR: Castalia Press.
Reid, J. B., Hinojosa-Rivero, G., & Lorber, R. (1980). *A social learning approach to the outpatient treatment of children who steal*. Unpublished manuscript, Oregon Social Learning Center, Eugene, OR.
Scarr, S. (1985). Constructing psychology. *American Psychologist*, *40*, 499-512.
Schaefer, E. S. (1965). Children's reports of parental behavior: An inventory. *Child Development*, *36*, 413-423.
Spanier, G. B. (1976). Measuring dyadic adjustment: New scales for assessing the quality of marriage and similar dyads. *Journal of Marriage and the Family*, *38*, 15-28.
Stouthamer-Loeber, M., Schmaling, K. B., & Loeber, R. (1984). *The relationship of single parent family status and marital discord to antisocial child behavior*. Unpublished manuscript, University of Pittsburgh, Pittsburgh.
Susman, E. J., Trickett, P. K., Ianotti, R. J., Hollenbeck, B. E., & Zahn-Waxler, C. (1985). Childrearing patterns in depressed, abusive, and normal mothers. *American Journal of Orthopsychiatry*, *55*, 237-251.
Walle, D. L., Hobbs, S. A., & Caldwell, H. S. (1984). Sequencing of parent training procedures. *Behavior Modification*, *18*, 540-552.
Willie, C. V. (1967). The relative contribution of family status and economic status in juvenile delinquency. *Social Problems*, *14*, 326-334.
York, P., York, D., & Wachtel, T. (1984). *Toughlove solutions*. Garden City, NY: Doubleday.

Working with Families: Expanded Roles for Child Care Practitioners

Karen Vander Ven

ABSTRACT. This paper describes various roles that professional child care practitioners can have in their work with families. The paper reviews changes in child care which increasingly necessitate work with families. Theoretically, the paper emphasizes how the family approach can be integrated with ecological and systems perspectives, how preventive approaches can involve families, and how parents can be involved in a variety of educational and therapeutic programs.

I see my role as adult, parent, peer and therapist. It is interchangeable. It depends on the situation, on the child, on anything.

Child care worker (Rathbun et al. 1981)

Child care workers are therefore increasingly finding themselves working with parents to help the parents learn how to be more effective with their children, rather than working with children themselves . . . it seems apparent that this will be a major part of the job in the future.

Jerome Beker (1973)

Karen Vander Ven is affiliated with the Program in Child Development and Child Care, School of Social Work, 1717 Cathedral of Learning, University of Pittsburgh, Pittsburgh, PA 15621. Grateful acknowledgement is made to the Research Fund of the School of Health Related Professionals, University of Pittsburgh, for support of the initial research for this paper.

Consideration of the role of child care practitioners in work with parents and families surfaces two paradoxes:

- that the *raison d'être* of child care workers to provide caregiving to children whose parents have been unable to has historically excluded them from working with these parents, and
- that while caregiving has been considered to be the basic socializer of children, the parents and child care workers whose role is to provide it and who have the closest and longest daily contact with children, have had the lowest status in society and in the service delivery system.

In recent years, however, this situation has begun to change. The earlier exclusion of child care workers from contact or work with children's families has been superseded by their beginning assumption of a variety of parent and family-oriented interventions.

Similarly, while child care still has a long way to go in achieving professional status, great strides have been made in recent years in that direction, so that *caregiving*, the joint function of families and child care workers, is increasingly valued as a core function in promoting positive human development. In line with this, parents are regarded more as partners with professionals than as passive recipients of professional services.

In view of these occurrences, the time seems appropriate to formulate a model for the role of professional child care practitioners in work with families, with a particular emphasis on identifying the social and theoretical sources that shape it, along with future trends that will precipitate further demands for it to be carried out. Thus, this paper will present:

- A review of the factors that converge today to shape the field of child care, and family characteristics that can be addressed by child care practitioners.
- A proposed model for parent and family work in contemporary child care practice based on guidelines generated by the review.
- Recommendations for enhancing the roles of child care workers with families in the future.

FACTORS SHAPING CHILD CARE AND FAMILY CHARACTERISTICS TODAY

For the purpose of conceptualizing the model for expanded roles of child care workers with families, the following areas seem relevant for review:

- The social context and attitudes that have shaped the structure and content of services.
- Changes in theoretical orientations underlying human services.
- Advances in the professionalization of child care.
- Established and emerging activities in child care practice with families.

Social Context and Attitudes Shaping Services

Prior to the 1960s the human service system pervasively blamed parents for problems they experienced with their children, as exemplified by Whittaker's "Family Etiology Hypothesis" (1976) and numerous personal accounts of parents' treatment by professionals, e.g., Wilson (1968), Spungen (1983). The need for parental support programs was not yet recognized and families were excluded from participative roles in interventions provided for their children.

The social upheavals of the sixties incisively changed this situation and there was a major movement towards the development of parent education, parent involvement, and parent participation programs.

This occurred first in early childhood programs such as Head Start, and later in programs serving exceptional children. Because residential programs were originally designed to "neutralize or inactivate a parent-child relationship" (Mayer, 1959), rather than to strengthen it, concepts of parent participation moved more slowly into this sector.

Today, the decline of the nuclear family and the emergence of a variety of alternative family structures, along with the solidification of a variety of modes of parent participation, supports the expansion of child care practice into work with families.

Theoretical Perspectives Affecting Services for Children and Families

The theoretical underpinnings that shape services to children and families have also changed over the years, with resultant implications for child care practice with families. The most relevant concepts are:

- *Ecology/Systems*. This embraces the notion that the most effective interventions delivered to children must impact not only their immediate environment, but a hierarchy of settings and systems that also exert an influence on them (Bronfenbrenner, 1975).
- *Interactional Theory*. Recognition of constitutional factors in human development (Chess, Thomas and Birch, 1984) suggests that characteristics of children, as well as parental practices and other environmental variables, jointly interact with each other to influence development.
- *Prevention and Health Promotion*. Conducting interventions either to head off future problems, i.e., prevention; or to directly promote skill and competence in dealing with the environment, i.e., promotion; are strong paradigms in today's human service delivery system.
- *De-Institutionalization*. This is the practice of moving people out of remote, larger institutions to provide care in community settings or the child's own home. Because it brings children, child care practitioners and children's families into closer interaction, it has major implications for child care practice with families.
- *Self-Help and Client Participation*. The emerging concept that persons with special needs can help themselves, utilize support systems and networks (Garbarino, 1982) and actually may participate in designing and delivering these services similarly is germane to structuring the role of child care practitioners with families.
- *Development as an Organizing Paradigm*. Psychoanalysis, behaviorism and cognition have been previous shapers of services; today development itself seems to be assuming this role.

The notion of encouraging positive development throughout the life cycle, fueled by the recent interest in adult development and meeting needs of the elderly, is gaining momentum and again has obvious implications for child care practice with children and families.

Professionalization of Child Care Workers and the Child Care Perspective

In the last 30 years, the organizing field of child care has made great strides in not only becoming more professionalized and recognized as providing an important service, but also in beginning to carve out a special and legitimate role in family work.

Training and Education for Child Care Practice

Although the earliest child care workers indeed spent the most time with the children, they were also the most poorly prepared for the task, as well as receiving little recognition for their importance. They were protected from having contact with parents, who were seen as the concern of other disciplines, particularly social workers. Child care workers themselves, usually in the field as an "interim" occupation, did not aspire to working with parents anyway. Youthful workers' rescue fantasies focused their attention on children themselves and how they could save children from their parents' inept ways; child care workers along with others were active participants in the "blame parents" mentality of the times.

In the seventies came organized activity towards professionalizing child care: a growing number of programs in higher education offering child care curricula, journals, conferences. Separate arenas in the field, e.g., early child education, day care, residential and day care and treatment, etc. began to recognize commonalities, suggesting a generic base for the practice of professional child care. The Conference-Research Sequence in Child Care Education produced *Principles and Guidelines for Child Care Personnel Preparation Programs* (1982) which included parent and family work in recommended curriculum content. These activities all surfaced interest in the concepts of expanded options for child care workers with various client populations.

The Child Care Worker as Life Space Integrator

The domino effect of the early eighties (Vander Ven, 1986), in which recent economic cutbacks in human services have eliminated some of the most highly compensated professionals, has encouraged the elevation of prepared child care workers to positions of greater clinical responsibility to replace those functions lost. A growing movement from the child care worker as "low man on the totem pole" to the child care worker as the *central* person in the team effort (Barnes, 1985; Peterson and Brown, 1982; Krueger, 1984). In this concept, the person who lives most closely to the children is the one who can best serve as the integrator of all other services that impact the child, so that s/he experiences the program as cohesive and meaningful. Because parents obviously are part of the child's life experience, they would fall within the child care practitioner's purview.

Personal and Professional Development for Lifelong Careers in Child Care

With the increase in professionalization in child care has come a concern with encouraging awareness of lifelong career opportunities in the field, not only to reduce the well-known frequent turnover of personnel, but to allow the development of an increasingly knowledgeable and skilled cadre of personnel capable of performing increasingly more complex functions. Since this latter process can only occur over time, career path options needed to be identified, along with the attributes required to be able to follow them. One such career path model has been described by Vander Ven (1980, 1981). Based on the premise that career development is accompanied by ongoing personal development as adults, these models include functions for child care practitioners in work with families.

The concept of personal and professional development as related to expanding functions of child care practitioners in work with families will be pivotal in the model to be developed later in this paper. The following *levels of practice*, referring to the degree to which practitioners' personal and professional development permits them to assume increasingly complex roles in parent and family work, will be utilized as a conceptual framework for the proposed model for expanded roles for child care workers in work with families.

This refers to the degree to which the practitioners' personal and professional development and maturity permit them to assume increasingly complex roles and responsibilities in child and family work.

– *The developmental/educational orientation* in child care practice focuses on direct client interventions at the behavioral level, and in general on the "here and now" of a situation, although the interventions definitely achieve long-term goals. Direct line, primary child care is intended to reflect application of the developmental/educational orientation, in which the purpose is to help clients—children or adults—best deal with reality, by developing appropriate skills for understanding and handling life's various encounters. Helping a child handle a temper tantrum by reviewing its immediate causes, demonstrating to a parent how to introduce an activity to an exceptional child, are examples.
– *The systems/ecological orientation* in child care practice focuses on "indirect" or contextual aspects of practice, in which services are delivered to the systems containing children and families, in order to make them more responsive and supportive. These activities include agency administration, staff supervision, community resource development and outreach program design, implementation and evaluation, training and education, advocacy, etc.
– *The therapeutic orientation* focuses on in-depth, dynamic factors in development; interventions may involve interpretation, review of historical events, and dealing with transference aspects. Since these elements are associated with traditional psychotherapy, child care practitioners in general have not embraced a directly therapeutic *process* in their work (although all their activities lead to therapeutic outcomes). With the domino effect and the increased longevity of prepared child care workers, some advanced practitioners are now adding the

therapeutic orientation to their skills within the framework of the child care perspective and thus this emerging role needs to be considered in a progressive model.

The Child Care Perspective

The most important outcome, perhaps, of the professionalization movement in child care is the refinement of what might be called the "child care perspective": that is, those activities and interventions that together *differentiate* the child care field from other human service professions. As child care practice logically expands into family work, this is the particular cadre of services that child care practitioners will be able to contribute.

The goal of child care practice is, briefly, to foster positive development in clients served, particularly through delivering various levels and forms of caregiving informed by the "child care perspective."

The "child care perspective" embraces utilization of:

- The self and one's behavior as a model for handling activities and situations in daily living.
- Interpersonal, communication and relationship-building skills within a life space context.
- Group process in the service of facilitating the development of all.
- Informed, developmental oriented caregiving through activities of daily living.
- Means to empower clients to effectively utilize community resources.
- The milieu or life space, including the physical environment, as an arena for keeping clients safe and nurtured, and for practice and delivery of interventions.
- Creative, educational, recreational, prevocational, expressive and other activity media as tools in delivering interventions.

Previously Established Forms of Professional-Family Interface

As the model for expanded roles of child care practitioners in work with families is to be derived from previously established modes of professional-family interaction, these will be reviewed.

The basic models for parent and family activation seem to have been established first in the early childhood sector. These include:

–*Parent Education*: providing information to parents, often in a preplanned form, to aid them in responding appropriately to their children's developmental needs.
–*Parent Involvement*: having parents serve on policy boards, provide administrative support services, and a variety of similar activities in which parents provide program input.
–*Parents as Interventionists*: Utilizing parents as co-workers or even co-therapists in the development or treatment of their own children.
–*Parent Advocacy*: Organizing by groups of parents, often of exceptional children, to advocate for services needed. Often such groups have been more effective in achieving results than professionals.

With the recognition that parental linkages with residential programs resulted in children's better social and cognitive progress (Seidl, 1984), parent programming finally began to emerge in the residential sector, sometimes involving child care workers.

The progressive Walker School had child care workers participate in meetings with parents to discuss concrete issues around the children and ways of managing daily problems (Hammond, 1973). McClintock (1975) describes a way in which parents, child, and child care worker met together in a problem-solving approach to resolve a specific crisis. In another program, child care workers worked collaboratively with other staff to provide a five-day-a-week residential program combined with two days at home (Astrakhan, 1975). Bertcher (1973), in a seminal paper, highlighted the power of child care workers as role models who could be effective in demonstrating to parents positive ways of managing their own children. And, indeed, some residential centers began to bring child care workers into discussions with caseworkers, in which the child care workers would describe how they handled tantrums, aggression, and other behaviors in the milieu. Other settings actually had parents come in to view workers on the job.

A PROPOSED MODEL FOR EXPANDED ROLES OF CHILD CARE PRACTITIONERS WITH FAMILIES

A review of the content just presented suggests that the following concerns should be addressed in designing a model for child care practitioner work with families.

Social Context

- Parents should be regarded as collaborators as much as possible.
- Parents need empathic, rather than "blaming" responses from professionals.
- Support activities should be provided to parents.
- Work with families requires attention to a variety of alternative family structures.

Theoretical Perspectives

- Family approaches should be ecologically and systems focused.
- Interventions should focus on characteristics both parents and children bring to their relationship, not just children alone.
- Activities with families should focus on health promotion and prevention, e.g., generally foster positive development in contrast to addressing specific difficulties or pathologies.
- Family interventions by child care practitioners will be delivered in a variety of settings: institution, community, and home.
- Targets of family interventions will increasingly include multigenerational populations.
- *Facilitating development*, as a core function of informed child

care practice, will be an increasingly recognized function in human services.

Professionalization of Child Care Workers

- Generic practice skills of the field will undergird child care practice with families, and will be included in child care preparation programs.
- Child care practitioners will assume integrative roles in service delivery, which by definition will involve parents and families.
- Ongoing personal and professional development of child care practitioners will empower them to perform expanded roles in work with families.
- The level of personal and professional maturity of practitioners is related to the complexity of roles that can be assumed in family work.
- The "child care perspective," the particular configuration of services offered by child care practitioners, is the basis for extension into family work.

Level 1: Direct Work with Children/Children and Parents

In Level 1 child care work, practitioners in general are youthful (between age 18-25), and are not yet parents themselves. The current functions of most workers at the entry level are to deliver primary service to children; however, program shifts as already described are increasingly requiring that entry level, and certainly more experienced direct line workers interface with parents as well. Developmentally, many young workers are not completely suited for parent work. Lack of complete separation from their own parents, strong identification with children, tendencies towards linear thinking are all variables contributing towards espousement of a "blame" and a lack of orientation towards interacting with parents (Vander Ven, 1980, 1983). Still, the shifting nature of programs is providing many opportunities for direct line workers, particularly as they progress beyond the entry level, to work with children and parents both.

At this level, the developmental/educative approach, as previously described, is appropriately applied in the following activities.

Information Giving

This can take two forms. In one, the worker *gives information* to the parent, particularly at times when there is an exchange of primary caregiving responsibility, such as when parents come to pick children up. This information may include behavioral observations, descriptions of the child's activities, reports of the child's progress, suggestions for handling a particular situation, etc. In the other, the worker frames information in a developmental context, e.g., "it's normal for children to not want you to leave; many others of Jimmy's age act that way" or in a managerial frame: "Perhaps tell him he has to go to his bedroom but doesn't have to go to sleep."

Management Modeling

This is a particularly valuable, although frequently underplayed, role for the skilled primary child care worker, and its reflective of the similarities between the parental and caregiver role. In this mode of practice, the worker models or demonstrates developmentally sound and behaviorally effective ways of handling day-to-day situations and activities. Management modeling has been, and can be further utilized, as a planned adjunct to parental services delivered by another discipline (e.g., social casework). It can also be a fundamental component within a larger activity, for example, child care work in the home which the general program format, in line with the developmental/educative approach, may involve joint activity sessions with child and parent, but also include management modeling. The power of management modeling as a particular service highly suited to child care workers to provide cannot be overemphasized.

Organized Parent Education

Organized parent group education is within the scope of the experienced child care worker, although to date this has been a less frequently utilized activity than some others. The fact that many of the approaches embodied in the *child care perspective* are highly appropriate to this form of family service supports the proposal that this role is one of those in expanded child care work with families. Focusing on developmentally based child management, activities, resource utilization and similar content, parent group education by the primary child care practitioner would involve developmental information giving in such areas as play, discipline, peer and sibling relationships, school, routines and activities of daily living, etc. Parent group education, in line with current trends, is one means of mounting preventive and (mental) health promotion activities.

The Child Care Practitioner as Collaborator in Parent Involvement

With the increase in parent involvement activities, child care practitioners on the line may find themselves working side by side with parents who have been assigned some form of on-line responsibilities. Since the child care practitioner is the stable person within this framework, it is important that s/he recognize the differences between the functions of parent support person and child care practitioner, as well as the ways in which the parent on-site can be optimally used. Application of the developmental/educative approach suggests that the practitioner use program design skills to enhance the effectiveness of the parent, as well as to prevent potential role conflict. Assigning the parent to specific children, areas or zones, or activities, may fall to the line practitioner, if not to his/her supervisor; under any circumstances the practitioner will have to recognize and constructively adapt to, the "dynamics" of such in-setting placements.

The Child Care Practitioner in the Family System

When considering the role of the primary practitioner in relationship to the families of children, it is crucial to consider the increasing emergence of child care workers into roles that successively approximate parental functions, within a home setting. These roles require that child care practitioners be able to operate smoothly within a family system. Unlike the child care worker with primarily programmatic responsibilities who, as previously mentioned, is likely to be a younger person, the age range in professional parent roles is more variable. Frequently mature people who have already raised their own families choose these roles.

Examples of these program models in which caregivers fulfill family and parenting roles are the generic or therapeutic foster parent (Gabor and Kammerer, 1982), the child care worker serving in a home-based setting (Herron, 1983), the American Nanny, the family day care worker or mother, respite caregiver, and the worker in the Teaching Family or Achievement Place model (Wolf et al., 1972).

In many of these models, the ability to interact smoothly with families around the joint concern of caring for the children; or to live compatibly within the family system, is as fundamental as that of working with the children. Therefore, the models comprise a significant component of the ways in which child care practice interfaces with families.

Level 2: Systems/Ecological Practice with Children and Families

In Level 2 of child care practice with families, practitioners have already spent a period of time in the field, often as primary care workers, and have received a promotion into "indirect" or contextual work as a supervisor, administrator, trainer/educator, or similar role. Sometimes these practitioners have by this time themselves become parents. This not only facilitates their movement into indirect roles, in which they must show concern for the functioning of other adults, but also their ability to identify with the concerns of *parents* and *families* as well as children. These more experienced and mature workers also have the ability to "think" in terms of systems, that is, multiple factors that may influence a particular situation.

The contextual/systems level of practice refers to the utilization of generic supervisory, training and administrative skills in meeting client needs through intervening in systems that impinge on them.

At this level, the contextual systems approach is appropriately applied to family-oriented practice in the following ways.

Information Giving

This is an expansion of the information giving role of the first level. The increased experience and background of practitioners allows them not only to deliver more sophisticated content, but also to package it in a way that educationally will make it more readily grasped and applied by the consumer. Practitioners at this level may be involved in giving information to parents and families through such means as newsletters, articles, media interviews etc. In more incidental contact with families, these practitioners can provide information on family support systems and ways in which families can maximally take advantage of them.

Role Modeling

At this level, there is still the option for the practitioner to serve as a role model. Since this person may have less direct contact with children, they may be models to both parents and direct line staff of ways of handling adult relationships and situations.

Designer of Parent Programs

The practitioner at this level may be involved in *conceptualizing* organized interventive programs for parents as well as actually delivering them face-to-face. Their structure and content would be shaped by relevant theoretical concepts, e.g., prevention, ecology. Such programs might include:

- Behavioral, developmental, or activity programs for parents to carry out with their children.
- Special parent participation programs, such as those previously described for parents of children and youth in residential programs.
- Home-based support programs, such as respite care, in-home parent support and education.
- Parent involvement programs, such as on-site or classroom participation, utilization of parent talents, parent assistance with special events, assistance to parents organizing for advocacy activities.

Organized Parent Education

Parent education by the Level 2 practitioner may embrace much of the same content as that described for Level 1: discipline, utilization of activities, etc. But the Level 2 practitioner now brings to this role contextual practice skills along with the knowledge and skills associated with the *child care perspective*, so that the *delivery* of the program is enhanced by use of more sophisticated educational and group leadership skills.

Integrator of the Child's Life Space

The child care practitioner in the role as integrator of the child's life space emerges at this level, utilizing special knowledge of child development and child care skills. In this function, similar to that of the case manager, the practitioner, with other team members, identifies, seeks, and coordinates a complete array of services needed to help a child and family reach developmental and treatment goals. Because of the obvious involvement of the family in the life of the child, and because of the movement towards family collaboration, a major function in this role is on activities pertaining to the family. In fact, the optimal use of the practitioner's role would be to help not only the child, but also the family, experience various interventions as an integrated, meaningful whole. This role is a complete reversal of the traditional child care worker placement at the bottom of the staff hierarchy and makes him central to a team effort, not peripheral to it.

Level 3: Advanced Therapeutic Work with Children/ Children and Families

Practitioners proceed to this stage with the prerequisites of extensive direct experience and clinically oriented educational preparation which qualifies them to utilize their special expertise around *children* in delivering service at a more in-depth level. Although there may not be a large number of child care practitioners at this level, observation indicates that there definitely are some; and the child care practitioner in a traditionally therapeutic role is becoming increasingly legitimized. The "domino effect" is a contributor to this phenomenon. Special communication skills in working with children and parents together are crucial to avoid overidentification with either party (Anglin, undated), and it undoubtedly requires the most professionally mature practitioner at this level to successfully relate to the bond between parent and child.

Among the services appropriately performed by practitioners at this level are:

Child-Oriented Family Therapy

Here, the practitioner may meet with child and family together, with the focus being more on the child than traditional family systems therapy. Given the fact that family therapy can ignore important attributes of the child (McDermott and Char, 1974), this approach, ideally utilizing the practitioner's expertise around children, provides important balance.

Dynamically Oriented Parent Education

Here a parent education model is used to frame consideration of child and family dynamics that may transcend the behavioral level; historical factors may be considered, interpretations provided; or media and methods used that will surface deeper issues and concerns. An example is the use of expressive media with the verbalization of childhood memories the experience evokes.

Special Approaches

There are a variety of special approaches that can be appropriately mounted by a clinical practitioner at this level. One example is that of *family play therapy* which is an "eclectic technique, combining elements from play and family therapies in addition to the methods of adult education. This technique includes parent(s), child(ren) and a therapist together in a pre-planned play situation" (Griff, in Schaefer, 1983, p. 65). Among the assets of this approach are the facilitation of application of recommended child management, communication, and interaction strategies by parents. Parents who have seemed "resistant" have seemed to thrive and to demonstrate significant changes as a result of participation in this modality. Family play therapy allows the therapist to serve as a role model, provides a more nonthreatening environment than talking therapy, shows the importance of play as a primary tool in enhancing development and communication, and encourages active problem solving.

Issues in Child Care Practice with Families

The compatibility between the child care perspective as provided by child care practitioners, and needs of children and their families that can be met by extension of that perspective into direct service to the child-family unit, is obvious. Yet there are some crucial issues that must be recognized as such approaches are mounted; the very close relationship between child care practitioners' functions and those of parents themselves can pose problems if not addressed.

Child Care Workers and Their Own and Children's Families

Because child care workers, like most people, have grown up in families, they may undertake child care practice with strong perceptions about the role and meaning of families to children and youth.

Younger child care practitioners often actually select the field because they are strongly identified with childhood (Vander Ven, 1980). Furthermore, they still may be involved with separating from their own parents. The result may be a strong tendency to reject or blame parents, as they think, in line with a characteristic rescue fantasy, "If only I could get this kid away from his awful parents and home—I could make him better!"

This issue might be called that of "the good and bad parent" in child care practice, following the psychological concepts of the all good, warm, nurturing parent; and the bad, rejecting, cold and rigid parent. In response, the novice practitioner will tend to see the child's parents as "bad" and themselves as "good." The "family etiology hypothesis" (Whittaker, 1969) often fuels the practitioner's pre-existing orientation towards creating a mental "good/bad parent" dichotomy between himself and the child's parents.

There are several concerns here. One is that this perception may encourage them to subtly downplay the children's real parents, despite Trieschman et al.'s (1969) astute observation that to do so is the "supreme insult," no matter how inadequate the real parents may be. The other is that the worker may encourage the child to actually see him as a "real" parent by actions which foster an overattachment of the child to the worker. This is a grievous error on the part of the child care worker, for it serves to develop fantasies in the child that the worker may indeed take the child in and become his parent. Because this is simply not going to happen, and because often the worker's relationship with the child is temporally limited, it is cruel of the worker to behave in a way that encourages or supports such fantasies. This is often the reason for agencies' policies against workers taking children to their own home.

Child care practitioners with children of their own need to grapple with issues surfaced by working with other children and their families. They may experience guilt if they feel that their time and energy investment in children outside their own family is excessive. If their own children have problems, even moderate ones, guilt and self-consciousness is compounded. Although more mature parent/practitioners can recognize that the determinants of children's behavior are complex – as already mentioned, a prerequisite for effective work with other parents – this is still a sensitive issue for them.

Child Care Practitioners as Substitute Parents

The issue of whether child care practitioners are "substitute" or "surrogate" parents is almost as old as the field itself. The issue is compounded by the fact that the role options for child care practice actually lie on a continuum in which one pole represents children and families treated as separate groups and in which the other represents the professional child care practitioner indeed serving a parental role. And, of course, the closer the parallel between the function of the child care worker and the child's real parents, – for example, when the child care practitioner is working within the child's home – the more acute the issue becomes. Statements such as "I care about this kid as if he were my own," and "I'm like a parent to him" reflect practitioners' perceptions of themselves as substitute parents.

Another manifestation of the "good/bad" parent dichotomy is in the tension that can often exist in child care or treatment programs between the child care worker as the substitute or "care" parent – the person who has the responsibility for daily care and activity, the therapist as the "transference" parent, and the agency director as the "power" parent (Mayer, 1959).

When child care workers have held low status in the treatment hierarchy, this has been detrimental to their potential to serve as effective role models for children, even though this is considered a basic function of child care workers. They are stronger role models if clients can see them receive rewards for the behaviors demonstrated (Bertcher, 1973); when workers receive little respect in terms of decision-making ability, their power as a role model is sorely diminished.

The Child Care Practitioner and Conjoint Child and Family Relationships

When child care practitioners interact directly with children and parents as a unit, the challenges increase, for they are now working within a larger, more complex system which requires that they must identify with the needs of both parties, as well as with the relationship between them. As Anglin (1984) puts it, the practitioner must relate to a *bond* or a *relationship*, rather than solely to an individual.

Working jointly with a parent and child poses the possibility of several dysfunctional relational patterns being followed: (1) relating solely to the child while excluding the parent (the easiest extension of the traditional child care practitioner role), thereby placing the parent in the position of relating to the bond between the child and the worker; (2) focusing on developing a relationship with the *parent* while de-emphasizing the child (possible particularly for older practitioners who, being parents themselves, are highly identified with the concerns of parenthood); and (3) forming a strong relationship with both parent and child without encouraging the relationship between the two of them. The appropriate stance is to relate to both child and parent, *and* to the bond between them (Anglin, 1984).

RECOMMENDATIONS FOR ENHANCING THE FUTURE ROLE OF CHILD CARE PRACTITIONERS IN WORK WITH FAMILIES

The analysis of historical contributors to the development of emergent roles of child care practitioners provided a logical rationale for the explication of the proposed model. For the components of the model to continue to come into its own a future orientation is required as well.

The following recommendations are made in support of advancing the future development of child care practice with families.

Training and Education

Perhaps the greatest need is for the legitimate establishment of family-oriented material in training and education programs for child care practitioners. The *Principles and Guidelines for Child Care Personnel Preparation Programs* (1982) recommends both curricular content and skills in family work. The following suggestions are more specific:

- *Adult and Life Cycle Development*. The expansion of contact of child care practitioners with persons of other age groups continues to occur whether or not the field formally defines itself as concerned with them. Practitioners encounter other adults not only as staff, but also as parents and older adults, e.g., in the growing number of intergenerational programs in child care settings. Thus, practitioners must know development throughout the human life cycle.
- *Family Dynamics*. Because of the large number of subtle issues around the relationship between child care practitioners and "real" parents, and the role overlap, child care practitioners must be made sensitive to family dynamics and family systems concepts, including the impact on families when an outside person enters their family system. This content should also cover expanded family systems, e.g., reconstituted families, multiple generation families, sibling relationships.
- *Staff Relationships Around Parenting Issues*. Practitioners at

all levels must be aware of the issues surrounding child care practitioners not only in working with parents and families, but also with other staff when the child care practitioner is fulfilling a parental type role.

– *Differences Between Roles of Parents and Child Care Practitioners*. Despite the role overlap between child care workers and parents, there are fundamental differences in their functions and practices, as is well articulated by Katz (1984). Articles such as this should be read and discussed in-depth by child care practitioners in training.
– *Theoretical Constructs*. The theoretical constructs initially discussed in this paper will continue to be salient in shaping family work and child care practitioners must be familiar with them, e.g., interactional theories of causation, basic temperament, ecology.
– *Contextual Practice Skills*. For advanced practitioners, all of the contextual or indirect practice skills facilitate the assumption of roles with families: program planning and design, teaching, team and group leadership, advocacy, communication.

Beyond the formal curriculum, there are several general stances that might be taken:

– Helping practitioners see how all aspects of the *child care perspective* can appropriately extend to work with adults, e.g., how activity programming and environmental design with children, and interpersonal communication skills, can be utilized in parent education.
– *Anticipatory socialization* activities to help practitioners be ready to assume more expansive roles in the future should be conducted, so entry level or preservice workers can see future opportunities for family work even if they are not yet developmentally ready to actually assume such roles.
– Offering of legitimate continuing education for advanced practitioners making the transition from behavioral to therapeutic modes of practice. Professional child care conferences have consistently offered workshops and seminars on various as-

pects of child care work with families (Austin and Vander Ven, 1985).

Professionalization of Child Care

Continued advancement in professionalization of the field of child care is essential for expanded roles. Perhaps the most compelling argument for this is the finding of Bertcher (1973) that role models with little power have little effect.

The concept of the child care practitioner as the logical *integrator* of the child's life space should continue to be pursued and developed. The child care perspective, with its emphasis on all of those contributors to a child's daily experience, including his family, underscores the appropriateness of this function. But since there are other disciplines that feel that analogous roles, such as case manager, are specifically within their purview, this will not be easy. An assertive stance, utilizing marketing strategies, will help child care practitioners feel comfortable in promoting this role as fitting for them.

Alignment with Emergent Trends in Family Life and Human Services

The field of human development and human services continues to need to respond to changing trends in overall society and in family needs and structure. Following are some that are particularly relevant:

–*Alternative Family Structures*. With fewer and fewer nuclear families, the need of such parent-child combinations as single parent families, reconstituted families, multigenerational families, teenage parents, working parents, etc., will increasingly require the services of family-oriented child care practitioners to fill in relationship and service gaps.

–*Family and Workplace Relationships*. There is a growing trend towards employers showing concern for family well-being as a means to heighten morale, and reduce turnover and absenteeism. On-site child care centers, parent brown-bag lunch discussion groups and many other kinds of programs are increasingly being developed. The family-oriented child care practitioner will be able to play key roles in helping employers design good quality, appropriately responsive program models.

– *Privatization*. The trend in health care towards self-employed service professionals is also gradually moving into child care, with the advent of private ownership of child care programs, and other child-oriented services. The increase in needs of working parents for a variety of services will maximize opportunities for family-oriented child care practitioners.

With the implementation of these approaches, the way should be paved for a legitimate expansion of child care practice into work with parents and families, which, because of its congruence with current needs and trends, should certainly improve service and quality of life for both the child and adult clients.

REFERENCES

Ainsworth, F., & Fulcher, L. (Eds.).(1981). *Group care for children: Concept and issues*. London: Tavistock.

Anglin, J. (1984, May). Education and support for parents: A challenge for group practice in the coming decade. Presented at the Conference Group Care Practice: The Challenge of the Next Decade. London: Kensington Town Hall.

Anglin, J. (undated). Counselling a single parent and child: Functional and dysfunctional patterns of communication. Victoria: School of Child Care, University of Victoria.

Anthony, E., & Benedek, T. (1970). *Parenthood: Its psychology and psychopathology*. Boston: Little, Brown.

Astrachan, M. (1975). The five-day week in residential treatment. *Child Welfare*, *41*(1), 21-23.

Austin, D., & Vander Ven, K. (1985). InterAssociation Child Care Conference: The first decade – Reflections on the advancement of the child care field. Unpublished manuscript.

Barnes, H. (1985, February). The child care worker as primary practitioner. *The Child Care Worker, 3*(2), 6-12 (Claremont, South Africa).

Beker, J. (1973). Editorial: Professional child care – Maximizing the impact. *Child Care Quarterly*, 2, 165-166.

Bertcher, H. (1973). The child care worker as role model. *Child Care Quarterly*, *2*(3), 178-191.

Chess, S., & Thomas, A. (1984). *Origins and evolution of behavior disorders: From infancy to early adult life*. New York: Brunner-Mazel.

Conference-Research Sequence in Child Care Education (1982). Principles and

guidelines for child care personnel preparation programs. *Child Care Quarterly, 11*(3), 221-244.
Curry, L., & Rood, L. (1975). *Heat Start handbook for parents*. Washington, DC: Gryphon House.
Featherstone, H. (1980). *A difference in the family: Life with a disabled child*. New York: Basic Books.
Gabor, P., & Kammerer, K. (1982). A meeting point: Developing treatment oriented foster care. *Journal of Child Care, 1*(3), 87-97.
Galinsky, E. (1984). How to work with working parents. *Child Care Information Exchange*, 1-4.
Garbarino, J. (1982). *Children and families in the social environment*. New York: Aldine.
Griff, M. (1976). Conjoint play therapy as a tool of the child care worker. Unpublished masters thesis, University of Pittsburgh, Pittsburgh, PA.
Griff, M. (1983). Family play therapy. In C. Schaefer (Ed.), *The handbook of play therapy*. New York: John Wiley.
Guerney, B. (1964). Filial therapy. *Journal of Consulting Psychology, 28*, 304-310.
Hammond, J. (1973). Child care workers as helpers to parents. *Child Care Quarterly, 2*(4), 282-284.
Herron, E. (1984). How to use your child care skills in the home. *Proceedings of the 1984 Interassociation Child Care Conference*. Sellersville, PA: Interassociation Child Care Conference, pp. 59-61.
Hobbs, N. (1974). Project Re-ED. In M. Wolins (Ed.), *Successful group care*. Chicago: Aldine.
Hough, R., & Stevens, J. (1981). Social networks as supports for parenting. *Young Children*, 50-60.
Jacobs, M. (1980). Foster parent training: An opportunity for skills enrichment and empowerment. *Child Welfare, 59*(10), 615-624.
Johnson, C., & Katz, R. (1972). Using parents as change agents for their children: A review. *Journal of Child Psychology and Psychiatry, 14,* 181-200.
Katz, L. (1984). Contemporary perspectives on the roles of mothers and teachers. In L. G. Kate (Ed.), *More talks with teachers*. Urbana, IL: ERIC Clearinghouse on Elementary and Early Childhood Education.
Lane, M. (1975). *Education for parenting*. Washington, DC: National Association for the Education of Young Children.
Littauer, C. (1980). Working with families of children in residential treatment. *Child Welfare, 59*(4), 225-234.
Magnussen, D., & Endler, N. (1977). Interactional psychology: Present status and future prospects. In Magnussen, D. & N. Endler (Eds.), *Personality at the crossroads: Current issues in international psychology*. Hillsdale, NJ: Lawrence Erlbaum.
Mayer, M. (1959). The parental figures in residential treatment. Paper presented at the Annual Meeting of the American Association of Children's Residential Centers, Chicago, November.

McClintock, D. (1975). Involving parents in solving a group problem in residential treatment: A case report. *Child Care Quarterly*, *4*(1), 44-47.

McDermott, J., & Char, W. (1974). The undeclared war between child and family therapy. *J. American Academy of Child Psychiatry*, *13*, 422-436.

Moreland, J., Schwebel, A., Beck, S., & Wells, R. (1982). Parents as therapists: A review of the behavior therapy parent training literature 1975-1981. *Behavior Modification*, *6*(2), 250-276.

Muir, K., Milan, M., Branston McLean, M., & Berger, M. (1982). Advocacy training for parents of handicapped children: A staff responsibility. *Young Children*, *37*(2), 41-46.

Peterson, R., & Brown, R. (1982). The child care worker as treatment coordinator and parent trainer. *Child Care Quarterly*, *11*(3), 188-203.

Powell, D. (1977). *The interface between families and child care programs: A study of parent-caregiver relationships.* Detroit: The Merrill-Palmer Institute.

Powers, D. (1980). Involving parents in therapy. In *Creating environments for troubled children*. Chapel Hill: University of North Carolina Press.

Principles and guidelines for child care personnel preparation programs (1982). *Child Care Quarterly*, *11*, 221-244.

Reisinger, J., Ora, J., & Frangia, G. (1976). Parents as change agents for their children: A review. *Journal of Community Psychology*, *4*, 103-123.

Schopler, E., & Reichler, R. (1971). Parents as cotherapists in the treatment of psychotic children. *J. Autism and Childhood Schizophrenia*, *1*(1), 87-102.

Seidl, F. (1974). Community oriented child care: The state of the art. *Child Care Quarterly*, *3*, 150-163.

Spungen, D. (1983). *And I don't want to live this life*. New York: Fawcett Crest.

Stevens, J. *Training parents as home teachers: A review of research.* Georgia State University: Department of Early Childhood Education.

Trieschman, A., Whittaker, J., & Brendtro, L. (1969). *The other 23 hours*. Chicago: Aldine.

Turnbull, A., & Turnbull, R. (1978). *Parents speak out*. Columbus: Charles E. Merrill.

Vander Ven, K. (1972). From raising kids to parenting: Current modalities of parent education. *Pittsburgh Area Preschool Association Publication*, *6*(2), 30-37.

Vander Ven, K. (1977). *Home and community influences on young children*. Albany: Delmar Publishing Company.

Vander Ven, K. (1980). A paradigm describing stages of personal and professional development of child care practitioners with characteristics associated with each stage. In *Proceedings of the Ninth International Congress of the International Association of Workers with Maladjusted Children,* Montreal.

Vander Ven, K. (1981). Patterns of career development in group care. In F. Ainsworth and C. Fulcher (Eds.), *Group care for children: Concepts and issues*. London: Tavistock.

Vander Ven, K. (1982). Educating practitioners in primary prevention. *Children in Contemporary Society*, *14*(2/3), 81-90.

Vander Ven, K. (1986). You've come a long way, baby; and you have a ways to go. In Competent caregivers: Competent children: Training and education for child care practice. A Special Issue of *Children in Contemporary Society*, *17*(3), 3-34.

Vander Ven, K., & Griff, M. (1976). Expanded roles for child care workers: Work with families. Presentation at InterAssociation Child Care Conference, December.

Vander Ven, K., & Griff, M. (1979). Expanded roles for child care workers: Work with families. Submitted to *Working Papers in Child Development and Care*. Victoria, BC: University of Victoria.

Vander Ven, K., & Mattingly, M. (1981). Action agenda for child care education: From settings to systems. *Child Care Quarterly*, *10*, 279-288.

Webster, C. D., Somjen, L., Sloman, L., Bradley, S., Mooney, S. A., & Mack, J. E. (1979). The child care worker in the family: Some case examples and implications for the design of family-centered programs. *Child Care Quarterly*, *8*(1), 5-18.

Whittaker, J. (1976). Causes of childhood disorders. *Social Work*, *21*, 91-96.

Whittaker, J. (1978). The changing character of residential child care: An ecological perspective. *Social Service Review*, *78*, 21-36.

Whittaker, J. (1979). Parents as partners in helping. In J. Whittaker (Ed.), *Caring for troubled children*. San Francisco: Jossey Bass.

Wilson, L. (1968). Journey of a lost boy. *Look Magazine*, February 6 and February 20.

Winkelstein, E. (1981). Day care/family interaction and parental satisfaction. *Child Care Quarterly*, *10*(4), 334-341.

Wolf, M. M., Phillips, E. L., Fixsen, D. L., Braukmann, C. J., Kirigin, K. A., Willner, A. G., & Schumaker, J. (1976). Achievement Place: The teaching family model. *Child Care Quarterly*, *5*(2), 92-103.

Woods, R. (1982). Learning to walk in a brave new world: Prevention and intervention with infants and families. *Children in Contemporary Society*, *14*(2/3), 35-42.

Yawkey, T., & Evenson-Bakawa, L. (1975). The child care professional-parent-child: An emerging triad. *Child Care Quarterly*, *4*(3), 172-179.

Family-Based Services: Preventive Intervention

Marvin E. Bryce

ABSTRACT. The value of family-based programs for the treatment and prevention of problems with children is increasing. The advantages of family-based programs is reviewed in terms of their general effectiveness and long-term cost. Much of the early work in family-based programs originated in the private sector but is moving into public programs as legislation and financial incentives support this approach. Ways of overcoming resistance and other problems in introducing family center programs in public agencies are discussed.

American society and the professionals and policymakers who reflect social values have traditionally affirmed the value of home and family as the basic institution. However, in practice the choice has been not so much to enrich and strengthen the family, as to supplant or replace it with out-of-home care. Reliance upon substitute care for the elderly, retarded, disturbed, delinquent, and neglected facilitated the removal of many children from their families, communities, and cultural heritage. Conditioned by past practice, limited in the capacity to conceptualize without extensive reliance upon familiar precepts, and fueled by unlimited funding, institutional and foster home placements were usually the first and often the only available resort for managing troubled children and youth well into the second half of the 20th century. Since 1910, institutional placements increased at twice the rate of population growth. Between 1961 and 1977, the number of children in foster care tripled while the total number of U.S. children declined (Dodson,

Marvin E. Bryce is affiliated with the Mississippi Bend Area Education Agency, 729 21st Street, Bettendorf, IA 52722.

1983). Once in the vast and uncoordinated system, exit was difficult and many children were stranded.

Problems created by prolonged separation from families were often deeper and more permanent than those that led to placement (Bryce, 1971; Gruber, 1978; Knitzer, 1978; Maas, 1959; Wolins, 1969). Turitz (1961) had tried to sound the knell when she urged that we free ourselves of traditional approaches and existing patterns of community and agency structure. However, as Stella Chess (1975) notes in a discussion of the New York longitudinal study on developmental theory, common knowledge is often denied or ignored by professionals. The same can be said of the business-oriented political policymakers who began to replace the human services professionals in 1961, about the same time governmental bodies began to embrace the concept that anyone could do social work.

This position led to the declassification or downgrading of requirements for child welfare workers, loss of status for the child welfare curriculum in schools of social work, and accompanying diminished skills and preparation to do child welfare work. Poorly trained child welfare workers became brokers for service, feeding children into established and powerful substitute care systems, primarily foster home and institutional care. The task force commissioned to study New York's child welfare system in the mid-1970s found it to be:

> . . . essentially a foster care system, despondently biased toward the long-term placement of children whose family environment had been disrupted. The reasons why the thrust of the system was directed toward foster care were many, but one, in particular, stood out. The primary reimbursement system for child welfare agencies, both public and private, was based on each child's stay in foster care at a more or less fixed per diem rate. This reimbursement formula all but dictated the traditional nearly complete reliance on foster care. (Pisani, 1982, p. 2)

While there had been numerous prior studies documenting the problem (Maas & Engler, 1959; Ricketts, 1959; Bryce & Ehlert,

1971; Vasaly, 1976; Keniston, 1977) which attracted the attention of astute and system-oriented individuals, none received the publicity and politicization comparable to research done in the late 1970s. Notable among the latter studies which helped prompt child welfare reform with increased emphasis on prevention include Vasaly's (1976) finding that half the children in foster care had received no service at home prior to placement. Also devastatingly critical of the child welfare system were the studies of Gruber (1978) and Knitzer (1978); analogous work in juvenile justice has been reported by Krisberg and Schwartz (1983) and Schwartz, Jackson-Beeck, and Anderson (1984).

Stimulated by the factors described above, Congress passed the Adoption Assistance and Child Welfare Act (PL 96-272) in 1980, creating unprecedented financial incentives for "placement prevention" and "reunification" programs to help children remain with their families. The Act clearly mandates family-focused child welfare services and suggests the need for a new system of social resources for families and communities. The Act's intent is to redirect federal fiscal incentives which until now have encouraged the separation of children from their families.

Succinctly, the primary factors providing momentum to the emergence of family-based preventive/restorative services are the following:

- Overwhelming documentation of deficiencies in the foster care system.
- The high fiscal, psychological, and social costs of behavior change sought by placement.
- Renewed recognition and application of the concept that when child development and human relationships are at issue, the family should be the service unit and the family's ecological system should be the service context.
- The advantages of avoiding, when possible, new risks which are introduced by placement and the disruption of continuity of environment and relationships, thus preserving whatever security the child may have.
- Public and professional concern for the many children who are

denied the benefits of a permanent home and are subjected to the trauma of multiple placements.

– Recognition that parents usually offer the greatest promise of permanency for their children and that permanency planning should begin at home.
– Accumulated evidence that many problems which lead to placement are more effectively, efficiently and humanely addressed in the context of the child's own family, community, and culture.
– Data pointing to the cost efficiency and service effectiveness of family-based preventive services.
– Legislative initiatives at both the state and federal levels which create financial incentives for family-based preventive services.

DEVELOPMENT OF FAMILY-BASED PREVENTIVE SERVICES

The emphasis in American culture on individualism, minimal government intervention, and cultural pluralism has contributed to the questionable assumption that families are served if people are served (Schorr, 1962, p. 457). The myth that family and government are completely separate entities has delayed the development of family-based preventive services. The Vanderbilt Institute for Public Policy (1977, p. 2) summarized the problem as follows:

> In the United States, the family has never been a major concern in the formation of public policy. In contrast, most other developed countries of the world have worked toward the family to take cognizance of its central role in the social structure. Nonetheless, families in the United States are affected by many public policies. What we have, then, is a family policy by default. . . . the nation has numerous policies that work against family solidarity and effectiveness and few policies that are designed explicitly to strengthen families. National programs have been launched that have had harmful effects on family life and child development; systems necessary for the

support of families and children have not been carefully worked out.

The concept that the family is the first line of defense for the prevention of the development of pathology, social deviance, economic hardship, physical and emotional harm and undue stress, is inherent in society. This axiom was a premise of the Elizabethan Poor Law. With the advent of child development concepts and psychological theory, astute observers began to recognize that in times of crisis and increased stress, the family becomes even more important to its members.

A child/family welfare system intended to preserve and strengthen the family and to provide permanency for children, must begin with policies, rules, attitudes, funding priorities, education and training programs, and expectations at every level of the bureaucracy, which favor and promote home-based, family-centered preventive efforts. While old values and practices still linger and dominate, recent new laws at both the federal and state levels are beginning to encourage practices designed to divert unnecessary placements of children. Some of these are discussed below.

The Pioneering Private Effort

Home-based prevention programs have evolved without benefit of standards, except those developed for individual programs. Programs vary in terms of types of families targeted, objectives, quality and intensity of service, staffing patterns, and commitment to the approach. Almost all of the early home-based, family-centered treatment programs were designed to provide an alternative to placement of one or more family members.

Primarily developed under private auspices, these programs focused on those families possessing a configuration of characteristics traditionally associated with out-of-home placement and where at least one family member was judged to be needing placement or to be at imminent risk of placement. Families were typically poor, single parent, and experiencing severe problems in three or more areas of family life. Generally problems had been present for several years and the families had received services from several community agencies. The families frequently seemed to be disenfranchised by medical, legal, educational, religious, and other established institutions (Bryce, 1978; Horejsi, 1981).

The St. Paul Family-Centered Project, the first home-based services program to mainstream intensive and modified social casework into the most problematic families and their environments, was initiated in 1950. The vital lessons learned from the project were not well disseminated (Birt, 1956; Overton & Tinker, 1957; Geismer 1958, 1960). The design of the project set out to test certain inter-related principles. The project workers related the success of the approach to aggressive outreach, which included the following:

1. The approach must be purposeful, related to a definite problem in the situation. It may be delinquency or truancy or other evidence of child neglect.
2. The approach should be open-minded: ready to hear and really understand the family's point of view.
3. It should be made with genuine confidence in the ultimate potential of each human being . . . (and) respect for human dignity.
4. It should be persistent. We must go often enough, stay long enough, go, despite rebuffs, discourtesy, frank hostility, and nonchalant denial of need or wish to use service. (Overton & Tinker, 1957, pp. 12-13)

Horejsi (1981, p. 22) notes some of the practical problems associated with the intensive home-based, family-centered approach.

> Implementation requires well-trained, confident, and highly motivated social workers. They must be able and willing to work many evenings per week, and perhaps for years, with a relatively small group of families. They must be able to cope with intense frustration, rejection, verbal abuse, and sometimes the threat of physical harm. An agency adopting this approach must justify a rather expensive program. Caseloads have to be small. Staff turnover must be kept to an absolute minimum. This is a program that must be built on long-term commitment; it is not something that you start one year and drop the next because of budget constraints. If you begin with the

> families, you must be prepared to go the distance. To begin and then drop these families is worse than doing nothing at all.

Horejsi also notes that this approach is not a substitute for adequate housing, income, health care, and education. Intensive home-based programs of more recent origin routinely apply much of what was practiced in St. Paul along with new techniques such as modeling, behavioral shaping, and family therapy.

Research indicates that 65% of the project families improved, and another 17.8% did not further deteriorate. These rather impressive results encouraged the public sector to field several projects with multi-problem families in ensuing years. However, these programs differed significantly from the St. Paul project and therefore the results were not encouraging (Geismer & Krisberg, 1967; Mullen, Chazin, & Feldstein, 1972; Wallace, 1963; Warren & Smith, 1963). Only the New Haven Improvement project, one of the more successful, reduced caseloads to 15 while the others maintained 30 to 50 cases. This, and other differences invalidates comparisons of results.

A number of intensive home-based prevention programs were spawned during the past two decades, again primarily by the private sector. The Home and Community Treatment program, funded by the Wisconsin Department of Health and Social Services system, was begun in 1969 as a component of the Mendota Mental Health Institute. The service was initiated because gains made with children in residential treatment were not being sustained after discharge, resulting in a high recidivism rate. Essentially, the staff extended the skills and techniques utilized in the institution, to the family, home and community. The program reports placement prevention for 90% of the client families (Cautley, 1980).

The Lower East Side Family Union in Lower Manhattan, New York, began a home-based prevention intervention program in 1972, in response to the continuing problems resulting from fragmented, nonintegrated, poorly coordinated, and therefore often unavailable services to families in the neighborhood. The program was initiated partly in response to the financial crisis faced by New York City and the discovery that the annual expenditure for substitute care was near $300 million for 29,000 children. The neighborhood settlement house was aware that many of the children and youth being placed were from very poor, primarily minority families. Existing programs simply did not relate to the need for comprehensive, accessible, coordinated services for these families. Dunu (1979, p. 211-224) and Weissman (1979) describe the background and structure of the program.

FAMILIES Inc., located in eastern Iowa, began its intensive home-based, family-centered service program in 1974, following the closing of one of the state's juvenile institutions. In the first two years of operation the agency served families in six counties with at least one child already dispositioned for institutional placement. Research indicates that 70% of those children served avoided placement (Bryce, 1978, p. 57). After the first two years, in response to pressure from referring agencies, services were expanded into three additional counties and families were accepted with children at imminent risk of any type of out-of-home placement, after which the success of placement avoidance increased to 91%. Iowa has reduced its foster care population by 45% in the past decade (Abigail, 1985, p. 21).

In 1974, Homebuilders in Tacoma, Washington, began an intensive family-centered service program. In the 119 families seen during the first two years of operation, Kenny (1977) reports that 188 family members were judged as having high potential for placement. Placement was prevented in 96% of the families through the third year of operation, and almost all of the cases reported continuing satisfaction with the resolution of the crisis which prompted referral.

Burt (1975), reporting on the final results of the Nashville Comprehensive Emergency Services Project, demonstrated how out-of-home placement can be reduced by the integration of services combined with the provision of comprehensive services to family units. Included in the findings were a 51% decrease in the number of children removed from home and an 85% decrease in the number institutionalized. The experimental program totally eliminated the institutionalization of children under six years of age and affected a significant decline in recidivism of cases. Follow-up efforts on those children who were placed and intensive work with their parents reduced long-term foster care (defined as two years or more) from 94% to 34% in that community (Hawkins, 1979).

Several family-centered preventive programs have been implemented by public agencies, either by counties or statewide, since the enactment of PL 96:272. More than 22 states have recently passed their own laws designed to enforce the requirements of the 1980 federal law. Additional states are considering similar bills (Abigail, 1985, p. 16). The government's refusal to define "reasonable effort" permits states who choose, to do little or nothing more than has been done in the past. In addition, the approach has been excessively diluted in some programs, in terms of intensity of service, and should not be compared to the exemplary programs described above.

Efforts in the Public Sector

Among the handful of states which have implemented exemplary intensive home-based prevention programs is Oregon. Its Intensive Family Services Program takes children only after a committee determines whether the child will be placed with a foster family or in some form of group care. Of the children in its study, 117 would have otherwise been sent into foster care. The remaining 95 would have gone into group homes (Abigail, 1985, p. 20).

New York, Colorado, Washington, Ohio and California are among the states which have attempted legislative remedies to the need for preventive services. Minnesota, Virginia, South Carolina, Iowa, and Utah are examples of states which have provided financial incentives or encouraged locally innovative prevention within the existing frameworks.

Public agencies have experienced difficulty adopting the approach for several reasons. These include the following:

1. Client assessment is keyed to services available in the agency, rather than the needs of the family in its environment.
2. Caseloads are frequently too large to permit workers to work intensively with families.
3. The organization of the public agency into specialized units, which emphasize protective and substitute care services, cre-

ates structural barriers to implementing significant family-centered prevention services.

4. Staff development programs focus primarily on training in agency procedures and offer little opportunity for workers to develop skills needed to work with the most troubled families.
5. The problems inherent in working with judges who are either unaware of or indifferent to the provisions in the Adoption Assistance and Child Welfare Act of 1980. In 1983 the National Resource Center for Child Advocacy and Protection of the American Bar Association found that, in many states which had not passed their own legislation mirroring the Federal Act, judges were uninformed about the new requirements. (Family focused law, 1983)
6. Untrained personnel. The Children's Defense Fund found that public child welfare workers started out underqualified and remained untrained. Many public agencies taught workers only how to complete forms correctly. The Children's Defense Fund emphasizes the tragedy and notes that well-trained social workers are the core of an effective helping effort. (Knitzer & McGowen, 1978, pp. 44-45)

Attempts by public agencies to include family-centered prevention services have been approached in much the same manner as protective services, adoption, and other services for "special" client groups. Family-based services are often added onto an already complex organizational structure and given status equal to the perceived importance of their particular constituent population. Family-based prevention programs have not achieved the recognition accorded child abuse and foster care programs in the service delivery system. The failure of the social service administration to view all of these constituent groups as part of the same fabric reflects an historical preference for serving the individual alone rather than as part of his/her family. The redesign of compartmentalized systems may be necessary in order to recognize the family as the principal client.

Another significant delay in the development of substantial preventive services has been the failure of funding agents to define more precisely the term "prevention." In its broad context, prevention refers to avoidance or prevention of something, anything. Sometimes the term is used to describe a type of family separation, as in "prevention of child abuse and neglect" (by placement) or "prevention of foster care drift' (as in permanency planning).

Home-based family-centered service as a method of intervention was originally designed to prevent unnecessary placement of children away from home. To be functionally meaningful, the term must be attached to another to form a phrase which denotes intent, i.e., "placement prevention." Many of the traditional, partial, or "band-aid type" services may indeed be preventive in nature. A homemaker, a visiting nurse, or a weekly appointment at the Mental Health Center is rarely adequate for a multiproblem family with a child in danger or at imminent risk of placement. Hoffman (1979, p. 11) noted this proclivity at the First National Symposium on Family Based Services at The University of Iowa:

> Our approach to the problem of our times has been fragmented and of the "band-aid" variety. At best, our current efforts can be described as small. True, the task is nearly overwhelming: but somehow, in some way we must turn ourselves around from our parochial way of operating.

In the public agency the current system of categorical services disperses clients in a relatively systematic fashion. For example, if a protective services worker is overburdened with cases, it is possible to place the children of particularly problematic cases in foster care, transfer the entire case or the child's case alone to the foster care worker, thereby relieving the protective services workers of responsibility. Although another case is likely to be assigned to the worker immediately, the movement of cases has a psychological effect for both the worker and agency. In addition, the movement of cases from unit to unit within the agency gives the appearance that client problems are being resolved. As Kadushin (1978) notes, service is too often fragmented, poorly coordinated vertically and horizontally, and discontinuous. He calls for integration of the organization.

Intake in the public agency is a critical function. Hutchison et al.

(1983) have proposed an intake system designed to facilitate service integration and focus on the family as the client.

FAMILY-BASED PROGRAM MODELS

Three models for the provision of family-centered prevention services are suggested. These include:

1. The Generalist-Specialist Family Service Division, which is an alternative to categorical services for children, adolescent parents and adolescent status offenders.
2. The Intensive Family Services Unit, designed to serve those families at greatest risk of imminent dissolution.
3. The Purchase of Service Model which is designed to serve high risk families, but is purchased from private agencies.

All three of the proposed models provide service in the home, focus on the family as client, and allow flexibility of intensity of service based on each client family's needs. In the same work the authors also propose a system for the classification of family needs as described below.

Transient needs pertains to families stranded for whatever reason in the agency's service area and who require minimal assistance to move on to their destination. It may also include casework services to migrant workers who pass through the agency's service area seasonally. Services provided by the agency are at a low level of intensity of total hours required to meet the family's needs. Coordination of community resources with advocacy and follow-up activities may be the focus of casework intervention. It should be emphasized that families are classified "transient" by their own definition. If the family members become permanent residents in the service area, the service requirements may change.

Emergency needs pertain to families whose difficulties are immediate, catastrophic, and are likely as not provoked by environmental factors beyond their control. The level of service required is intense and of short duration. The resources required are likely to be found in the community, rather than in the agency itself. Therefore, the agency response may be largely coordinative, e.g., identifying appropriate resources, coordinating and following up on their delivery, and advocating for community services in the family's behalf. Again, should it become evident that the family's situation requires more intensive service and the family agrees to continued involvement with the agency, another level of services may be assigned.

Limited-Situational needs characterize families who have begun a cycle of maladaptive interaction, which can be arrested by change in one or two areas of functioning. With concerted, time-limited efforts by the social worker and agency and community resources, they can regain their equilibrium and function independently again. The service level may be intense initially, but is likely to result in termination of services within a short time frame. Without appropriate intervention, families in this classification tend to continue the cycles of maladaptation which are then defined as additional problems, eventually requiring longer services or resulting in family breakup. This cycle can and should be broken by immediate intervention.

Multiple-Problem needs characterize families that exhibit a host of problems/needs, which may include child abuse and neglect. These families require numerous agency and community resources and should receive intensive family-centered services until their situation is stabilized. Families with multiple needs have been successfully treated by private agencies using family-based interventions and often show dramatic changes as a result of intensive service.

Maintenance needs pertain to families who exhibit numerous difficulties of a long-standing, perhaps multi-generational, nature. Although these families are small in number, they typically absorb a significant proportion of casework hours and agency resources. If these families fail to respond to intensive services, it might be reasonable to propose that the agency's resources are being overused with little hope of successful problem resolution. Therefore, family-centered services should be limited to maintenance efforts, providing only those services required to maintain the family at a minimal level of functioning, with the goal of forestalling out-of-home placement. Of course, a crisis situation may present new possibilities of change to the family, so the option of renewing intensive services must always remain open.

The degree of intensity of service by classification is illustrated in Figure 1.

It is suggested that a group of experienced child and family services supervisors review a randomly selected sample of active cases across child-serving units. Through group process, supervisors identify primary or root problem(s) that may be central to each family's difficulties and that can be addressed either directly or in coordination with other community services providers. Based on problems identified and group consensus, case are then assigned to either "Limited-Situation needs" or "Multiple-Problem needs" classification. The criteria used for assignment of cases to each classification is then identified and documented by the group.

Estimates of the total caseworker time required to address the social work needs of families by classification may also be made by the group. The resulting criteria and time estimates may then be used over time by the intake and family services supervisors to test their validity and utility.

The same methodology may be used to establish criteria for maintenance needs. However, this classification needs to be thought through carefully by staff specialists and the agency's administrators since the tolerance level of communities demanding active service interventions for certain families will vary.

Both the emergency needs and transient needs are self-defining,

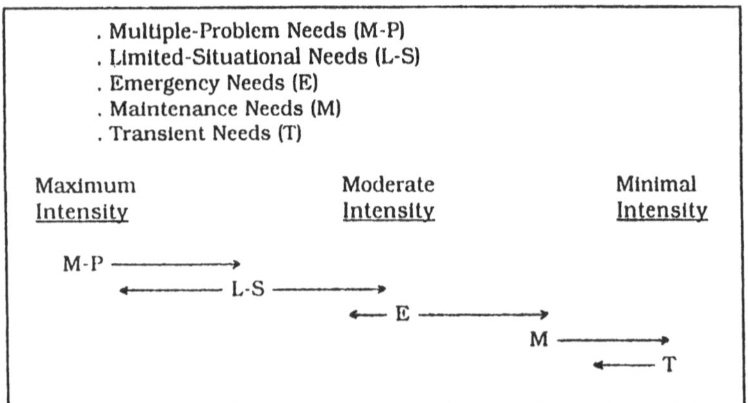

Figure 1. Degree of Intensity in Terms of Service Hours Expended.

and criteria for recognizing cases in these classifications should be relatively easy to construct.

Services in the five classifications are integrated into the service delivery system design. For example, the Generalist/Specialist Family Services Model is composed of two core components (intake and family services) and at least four core support services (day care, parent aide, foster care, and adoption) provided either directly by the public agency or purchased from private, voluntary agencies in the community.

ADVANTAGES OF PREVENTIVE SERVICES IN THE HOME

Doing treatment ("treatment" as used here means dealing with in a specified manner and is not to be construed in a medical sense) in the home offers a number of advantages. Perhaps the primary psychological advantage is related to the client's increased sense of personal control. Robert White's (1963) concepts of ego psychology seem applicable in this regard. White developed the notion that the primary drive in individuals is the drive to be competent in one's own life, and that when this drive is frustrated, the individual is deeply damaged. This phenomenon is being experienced today by many in association with the loss of job, the family farm or other family business. Under these and similar circumstances parents who have for many years been able to effectively control their destiny and that of their family, lose that power. Reactions to the loss of control include rage, withdrawal, acting out in protest, depression, suicide, and a keen sense of failure and decreased self-esteem. Agencies across the land are striving to help these families regain a sense of control over their destiny. Going to the family's home conveys respect and assures concern and caring. Clients feel more in control of the situation in familiar surroundings and more competent in controlling the interaction.

In the narrative evaluations done by the families in the St. Paul Family-Centered Project, families frequently referred to the importance of the worker coming to them; that it conveyed a sense of caring and concern (Compton, 1975). The families felt they had more control over what happened, and that they were of some worth. In a more recent study of 94 families who had received in-home treatment, the families valued most highly the fact that the home was the service setting and that the parents remained in charge of the family (Bryce, 1978, p. 56). As professionals we frequently fail to appreciate the physical and emotional difficulties that keep families from coming to the agency. In addition, many lack the trust to seek help, even though they may be desperate.

In-home treatment reaches more people. Some are terminally ill or severely handicapped; others are elderly or bedridden. Parents with infants or preschool children and families who cannot coordinate their schedules can be reached. Some people are without transportation, some are mentally ill, and others are geographically isolated and do not drive. From a systems perspective multigenerational members can be easily included in treatment. When indicated, significant neighbors can be included in family treatment sessions. Other advantages include the following:

1. Assessment and treatment takes place in and includes the family's home and community and the interrelationship of the family and its environment. Thus the adequacy of the community to meet the family's needs is also addressed.
2. "Being there" when the family experiences its greatest difficulties makes it possible for the in-home practitioner to observe first-hand the extent of mental, behavioral or physical imbalance between individual, family and community needs.
3. Reliance on second and third person reporting "about" an historical event is avoided and efficiency and accuracy of assessment and treatment are increased.
4. First person observation as a source of information is utilized. For example direct, formal, informal, and streams of behavior observations are part of the ongoing assessment, planning and treatment processes.
5. The ecological context makes it possible to view personal functioning in the social matrix of the family, and to treat it accordingly.
6. In-home treatment facilitates observation and intervention in the vital areas of organization, routine, rituals, home management skills, child management, and parent-child interac-

tion, thus going beyond merely giving directions or telling parents what to do.

7. Possibilities are expanded for programming firsthand for clients who may have low self-esteem, are lonely, for those who may not know how to play or recreate, or those who may be angry, anxious or depressed and will likely never see a clinician in the office.
8. The practitioner is afforded direct frequent exposure to the family and individual strengths, which often profoundly affects positive contagious attitudes and motivation, as well as decisions and treatment.
9. Being frequently present and available fosters the development of trusting relationships essential to treatment, and particularly to the nurturing/reparenting needed by some parents.
10. Theoretical perspectives, which may conflict, need not be a problem because the techniques are generally compatible. The inclusion of differing theories increases the chances that the needs in a given family and community will be addressed.
11. Common sense, intuition, and respect for the uniqueness of each "family in situation" takes precedence over theory and technique.
12. Staff time, skills and resources sufficient to assess, formulate and implement a service strategy relevant to the family's needs, is made available.
13. Being "in family and community" makes it possible for the in-home practitioner to assume a key role in assisting the family to develop a support system.
14. The practitioner, being close to the family and aware of the multiple forces impacting on it, is in a key position to coordinate services.
15. Psychological and concrete services are integrated.
16. In-home treatment allows a timely, immediate and intensive response to crises, thus serving an important preventive function.
17. There is minimal reliance on terminology which implies, or

has come to be associated with, hopelessness, e.g., schizophrenic, chronic, inadequate personality, character disorder.

Being in the home allows for a planned sequenced program of service with the parents in the primary role, where techniques are more easily applied, including didactic teaching, modeling, coaching, counseling, etc. Reliance on "telling" parents what to do is minimized. New behavior patterns cannot be expected to be stress resistant until they have become habitual. Being in the home allows for practicing, thus strengthening new behaviors.

Leverington and Wulff (1982) provide an interesting account of their experiences as home-based, family-centered practitioners. They point out the advantages of the heightened reality context, the presence and use of symbolism in the home and the opportunities to build upon strengths. They note that the worker can view the family differently and construct unique interventions. Chances for success are enhanced because high quality information is abundant, high levels of rapport are developed, and hope is increased as the worker relates to the total family about their many concerns.

FINANCIAL AND LEGISLATIVE SUPPORTS

Prior to the 1974 Social Services Amendment established under Title XX, federal legislation provided little financial incentive for preventive services. The act established a program of grants to states for social services, intended to include preventive service intervention, including home-based care. Unfortunately, the grants were utilized primarily to expand the substitute care programs. In the same year, the Juvenile Justice and Delinquency Prevention Act provided federal funds for alternatives to incarceration and for the identification, prevention and amelioration of child abuse and neglect.

Historically, one rationale for placement of children in institutions was to provide them with a special education program. The 1975 Education for All Handicapped Children Act (PL 94:142) encourages a free, appropriate education in the least restrictive setting feasible, for all handicapped children. This makes it possible for many children to remain in their homes. However, it also places additional demands on local service agencies because many of the families are in need of therapeutic services.

Nowhere has the failure to recognize and appreciate the importance of culture and the power of family and clan relationships been more clearly demonstrated than in the experience of the Native American. Byler (1977) describes the placement of 25% of American Indian children away from family and tribe as perhaps the most destructive and tragic aspect of American Indian life today. The Indian Child Welfare Act passed in 1978, was designed to encourage alternatives to unnecessary and inappropriate placements of Indian children. The home-based approach and philosophy are compatible with the intent of the Indian Child Welfare Act and the desires of Native Americans to preserve the integrity of Indian family life and traditions.

At the state level of government a number of funding strategies have developed. Iowa, in 1974, closed one of the state's institutions for juveniles and utilized the funds for noninstitutional alternatives. Home-based, family-centered services were purchased by the Department of Social Services from a newly created agency (FAMILIES, Inc.) serving nine counties in Eastern Iowa. With consultation and training by the FAMILIES staff, another home-based, family-centered service agency was created (FAMILIES, NEI) to expand the service, and existing traditional family and child welfare agencies, including some which previously offered only residential and/or foster home care, added a home-based, family-centered service unit. Most of the state's 99 counties now have access to home-based, family-centered services. Unfortunately, as with other social services nationally and in Iowa, the home-based, family-centered services effort has been significantly curtailed by the critical economic situation.

In 1976 California passed the California Family Protection Act in an effort to reform an expensive and ineffectual foster care system. Implementation was piloted in two counties. Influenced by the 1974 Juvenile Justice and Delinquency Prevention Act, Washington State passed its Alternatives for Incorrigibles legislation (SB3116) in 1976. This legislation was followed by HB371, which stated that maintaining the family unit should be the first consideration in all cases of state intervention into children's lives. In 1979, Colorado enacted legislation capping state foster care expenditures and the rate of state reimbursement to counties for foster care. This encourages counties to utilize or create alternatives to placement. The law requires counties that utilize state foster care funds to also create a placement alternative commission to develop alternative programs (Becker, 1980).

Pilot in-home service programs have been fostered by some states by the provision of seed money to counties. In Virginia, the Department of Social Services used federal child welfare (Title IV.B) funds to provide grants for preventive programs to counties. This approach facilitates community education regarding needs and promotes local leadership in program development. Increased commitment and comfort with nontraditional or preventive services are also encouraged.

Some states provide fiscal incentives for preventive services by altering the list of what they will reimburse. Those states provide fiscal incentives for preventive services and make reimbursement contingent upon compliance with the law. New York is an example. New York enacted Child Welfare Reform legislation in 1979, becoming the first state to mandate preventive services. The rate of reimbursement in the state for mandated preventive services is 75% and less for nonmandatory preventive services. While New York's fiscal commitment to preventive services exceeds that of other states, the state's expenditure for foster care for 1982 was more than ten times that for preventive services (Statewide Youth Advocacy, 1984, p. 2). Janchill (1981, p. 3) points out that costs are usually ascribed to payments made directly to providers of foster care and usually exclude local, state and federal expenditures for administration, supervision, accountability tracking, and computerized information retrieval systems. She notes that these administrative costs may exceed those for direct care.

The plan as implemented has not solved New York's heavy reliance on substitute care partly because private child care agencies continue to rely on substitute care solutions and those agencies have always been powerful influences in the child welfare industry in New York. In addition, "prevention" is loosely defined as is the case in the federal law (96:272) and no adequate system has been adopted for identifying families at greatest risk of placement.

New programs are vulnerable in times of economic retrenchment. In addition, bureaucracies are not easily altered and as Sosin (1979) notes, social mandates, legislation and laws are often ignored, evaded, or subverted. Even the best organized efforts with the most skilled people involved can fail if the statutory structure of the state does not allow recourse to new developments and techniques (Bryce & Lloyd, 1980).

COMPARATIVE COSTS: FAMILY-CENTERED PREVENTIVE SERVICES AND SUBSTITUTE CARE

Comparisons among programs reveal considerable differences in reported cost associated with service delivery. These variations may be attributed to factors such as duration and style of service, the number of casework hours expended per client family, salary differentials, staffing patterns, and accounting and data collection methods used.

Table 1 illustrates the range of expenditure per family and the

TABLE 1. Service and Cost Results: Intensive Family-Based Programs

Agency	Average Length of Service	Cost Per Family	Percent of Placement Prevention
Families, West Branch, Iowa	5 months	$4,000	91%
Homebuilders, Tacoma, Washington	6 - 8 weeks	$1,769	92%
Intensive Family Support, Hillside Children's Center, Rochester, New York	6 - 7 months	$1,338	88%
Oregon Intensive Family Services, Department of Human Resources, Children's Services Division, Salem, Oregon	90 days	$1,000	92%

percentages of children prevented from substitute care placement reported by four home-based, family-centered service programs.

Families Work, a component of Parkhurst Parent and Child Center in Schenectady, New York, conducted a pilot home-based preventive services program in 1980. The county Department of Social Services identified 506 children at high risk of placement. This finding, plus incentives in New York's 1979 Child Welfare Reform Act, prompted a search for alternatives to placement. The project was evaluated by Tavantzis et al. (1985, p. 75-88). They report a placement avoidance rate well within the 70-90% range reported by other home-based prevention programs. Referring agencies projected that of the 32 mandated youths seen in the first eight months, 13 would have been placed in foster homes, 12 in group homes, and seven in institutions, at a potential expenditure of $253,082 per year. (Children in foster care in New York exceed the national average length of stay of three years.)

The cost of *Families Work* was $35,290, plus $30,818 expended for youth who were placed after the program. The data is based on the assumption that each of the 32 children would have been placed for the entire period. Also, not included in the projections were costs of aftercare services, if any, following *Families Work* termination. However, the researchers report that if only three institutional placements had occurred, the cost would still have exceeded the cost of home-based services prevention.

Initial commitment of financial and staff resources for family-centered preventive services should be offset by savings and maintenance costs for foster and institutional care during the first year of a family-centered preventive program. Most family-centered service programs provide early assessment and intensive, time-limited service intervention in the early phase, with declining investment as the family becomes more functional. Closure generally occurs within three to nine months.

The primary difference between family-based services and foster care expenditures is placement maintenance costs. Since family-centered services initially call for a greater commitment of worker time and support services than foster home services, per client expenditures may be higher than family-centered services expenditures even when monthly maintenance costs are included. However, when projected substitute care costs are discounted over the average length of time a child is likely to remain in placement, family-centered services are more cost efficient. Often other children in the home are in greater pain than the one referred and work with the family unit in its context also benefits those children.

Cost efficiency of the home-based preventive approach is especially impressive when all of the family members who receive service are included in the calculation of costs per individual receiving service.

Data supplied by the division of social services of an East Coast state were subjected to a prospective analysis. An attempt was made to project expenditures and cost savings for children who were expected to enter the state's child welfare system in the ensuing year. No attempt was made to project savings to the agency from reunifying children who were already in substitute care with their families. Because the number of children expected to enter the foster care program in the coming year was unknown, estimates were based on the previous year's 2145 children who entered the state's foster care program. Sixty-seven percent (67%) went into foster family homes. Twelve and one-half percent (12.5%) went into institutions. The remaining 20.5% did not enter substitute care. It is assumed that the latter group returned home within a few days or were placed in free homes of relatives or friends.

In the analysis, the assumption was that by providing family-centered services at a level of effort commensurate with a given family's needs, a significant number of children could be prevented from substitute care placement when the value of the cost of family-centered services (as determined by worker salary and caseload to worker ratio) was subtracted from the benefits to the agency (as determined by the net value of maintenance expenditures over the average length of time a child remains in placement) the net benefits accruing to the agency could be determined.

After a rate of 10% was computed for dollars committed for placement for a period of three years, the average length of time a child remains in placement in that state, net benefits were $8,324,000 (Hutchinson et al., 1983, p. 67). It should be noted that costs for training or retraining workers and supervisors, essential for initiation of a successful home-based, family-centered service program, were not included.

CONCLUSION

Cumulated evidence indicates that home-based, family-centered prevention services are cost efficient and service effective. The decision to place a child outside his/her home is a monumental one to be made only with the greatest care and deliberation. This awesome responsibility too often is left to individuals who have inadequate resources for family assessment and preventive intervention, and to those who frequently underestimate the power of family attachments. If parents and children are attached at all, an intervention that does not empower the parents by working through them is effectively working against them (Tavantzis et al., 1985, p. 75). Just as every family potentially has available the resources of substitute care, each family, with informed consent, should have the option of home-based, family-centered preventive service (Bryce, 1981, p. 10).

REFERENCES

Abigail, N. (1985). *Keeping families together*. New York: Edna McConnell Clark Foundation.

Becker, M. (1980). *House bill 371: An introduction*. State of Washington: Office of Program Research. See also Revisions 17 & 18 to Manual G (2/80), Washington State Department of Social and Health Services.

Birt, C. (1956). Family centered project of St. Paul. *Social Work, 1*, 41-47.

Bryce, M. (1978). *Client and worker comparison of agency organizational design and treatment techniques in an intensive home-based social service program for families*. Iowa City, IA: University of Iowa, Doctoral thesis.

Bryce, M. (1980). Home-based care: Problems and perspectives. In M. Bryce & J. Lloyd (eds.), *Treating families in the home: An alternative to placement*. Springfield, IL: Charles C Thomas, 5-11.

Bryce, M., & Ehlert, R. (1971). 144 foster children. *Child Welfare, 9*, 499-503.

Bryce, M., & Lloyd, J. (1980). *Placement prevention and family unification: Planning and supervising the home based family centered program*. Iowa City, IA: National Clearinghouse for Home Based Services to Children and Their Families, University of Iowa.

Bryce, M., & Ryan, M. (1978). *Intensive in-home treatment: An alternative to out-of-home placement*. In J. Hanks (ed.), *Toward human dignity*. Washington, DC: NASW, 155-168.

Burt, M., & Balyeat, R. (1975). *From non-system to system: Evaluation of the comprehensive emergency service system for neglected and abused children*. Nashville: Burt Associates.

Byler, W. (1976). *The destruction of the American Indian family* (ed., S. Unger). New York: Association on American Indian Affairs. (See also W. Byler, Statistical survey of out-of-home placement of Indian children. New York: Association on American Indian Affairs.)

Chess, S. (1975). Development theory revisited. *Canadian Journal of Psychiatry, 24*, 101-111.

Compton, B. (1975). *The family center project revisited*. Iowa City, IA: National Clearinghouse for Home Based Services to Children and Their Families, University of Iowa.

Dodson, D. (1983). Preventive and reunification services. *Legal response: Child advocacy and protection*. Washington: American Bar Association.

Dunu, M. (1979). The lower east side family union: Assuring community services for minorities. In S. Maybanks & M. Bryce (eds.), *Home-based services for children and families: Policy, practice and research*. Springfield, IL: Charles C Thomas.

Fahl, M., & Morrisey, D. (1979). The mendota model: Home community treatment. In S. Maybanks & M. Bryce (eds.), *Home-based services for children and families: Policy, practice and research*. Springfield, IL: Charles C Thomas.

Geismer, L. (1960). *Measuring family functioning*. St. Paul: Greater St. Paul Community Chest and Councils.

Geismer, L., & Ayers, B. (1958). *Families in trouble*. St. Paul: Greater St. Paul Community Chest and Councils.

Geismer, L., & Krisberg, J. (1967). *The forgotten neighborhood*. New Jersey: The Scarecrow Press.

Gruber, A. (1978). *Children in foster care: Destitute, neglected, betrayed*. New York: Human Sciences Press.

Hawkins, R. (1979). Developing comprehensive emergency services. In S. Maybanks and M. Bryce (eds.), *Home-based services for children and families: Policy, practice and research*. Springfield, IL: Charles C Thomas, 103-111.

Hoffman, G. (1979). Turning ourselves around: A challenge to the professional community. In S. Maybanks and M. Bryce (eds.), *Home-based services for children and families: Policy, practice and research*. Springfield, IL: Charles C Thomas, 5-12.

Horejsi, C. (1981). The St. Paul family centered prospect revisited: Exploring an old gold mine. In M. Bryce and J. Lloyd (eds.), *Treating families in the home: An alternative to placement*. Springfield, IL: Charles C Thomas, 12-23.

Hutchinson, J., Bryce, M., Landman, M., Lloyd, J., & Nelson, K. (1983). *Family centered social services: A model for child welfare agencies*. Iowa City, IA:

National Clearinghouse for Home Based Services to Children and Their Families, University of Iowa.

Janchill, M. (1981). *Guidelines for decision making in child welfare*. New York: Department of Social Services.

Kadushin, A. (1978). *Child welfare strategy in the coming years*. Washington, DC: Children's Bureau.

Keniston, K. (1977). *All our children: The American family under pressure*. New York: Harcourt Brace Jovanovich.

Kinney, J., et al. (1977). Homebuilders: Keeping families together. *Journal of Consulting and Clinical Psychology, 45*, 667-673.

Knitzer, A., Allen, M., & McGowen, B. (1978). *Children without homes*. Washington, DC: Children's Defense Fund.

Krisberg, B., & Schwartz, I. (1983). Rethinking juvenile justice. *Crime & Delinquency, 29*, 333-364.

Leverington, J., & Wulff, D. (1983). *In home family therapy*. Iowa City, IA: National Clearinghouse for Home Based Services to Children and Their Families, University of Iowa.

Lloyd, J., & Bryce, M. (1980). *Placement prevention and family unification: A practitioner's handbook for the home based family centered program*. Iowa City, IA: National Clearinghouse for Home Based Services to Children and Their Families, University of Iowa.

Maas, R., & Engler, R. (1959). *Children in need of parents*. New York: Columbia University Press.

Mullin, E., Chazin, R., & Feldstein, D. (1972). Services for the newly dependent: An assessment. *Social Services Review, 41*, 4, 309-322.

Overton, A., & Tinker, K. (1957). *Casework notebook*. St. Paul: Greater St. Paul Community Chest and Councils.

Pisani, J. (1982). *The temporary state commission on child welfare: Final report of the chairman*. Albany: New York State Senate Report.

Ricketts, B. (1959). *Child placement and its effects on the child and his family*. Northampton, MA: Smith College, Master's thesis.

Schorr, A. (1962). Family policy in the United States. *International Science Journal, 14*, 452-467.

Schwartz, I.M., Jackson-Beeck, M., & Anderson, R. (1984). The "hidden" system of juvenile control. *Crime & Delinquency, 30*, 371-385.

Sosin, M. (1971). Social work advocacy and the implementation of legal mandates. *Social Casework, 60*, 265-273.

Statewide Youth Advocacy (1984). *Preventive services under the child welfare reform act: An advocacy perspective*. Rochester, NY.

Tavantzis, T., Tavantzis, M., Brown, L., & Rohrbaugh, M. (1985). In M. P. Mirkin & S. L. Koman (eds.), *Handbook of adolescents and family therapy*. New York: Gardner Press, Inc., 69-88.

Turitz, Z. (1961). Obstacles to services for children in their homes. *Child Welfare, 40*, 1-5.

Vanderbilt Institute for Public Policy Studies (1977). *The program for the center of families and children*. Nashville, TN.
Vasaly, S. (1976). *Foster care in five states: A synthesis and analysis of studies from Arizona, California, Iowa, Massachusetts and Vermont*. Washington: Social Research Group (George Washington University), DHEW Pub. No. (OH) 76-30097.
Wallace, D. (1963). The Chemung county evaluation of casework service to dependent multiproblem families: Another problem outcome. *Social Service Review*, *41*, 379-389.
Warren, R., & Smith, J. (1963). Casework service to chronically dependent multiproblem families: A research demonstration. *Social Service Review*, *37*, 33-40.
Weissman, H. (1978). *Integrating services for troubled families*. San Francisco, CA: Jossey-Bass.
White, R. (1963). *Ego and reality in psychoanalytic theory*. New York: International University Press.
Wolins, M. (1969). Group care: Friend or foe? *Social Work*, *14*, 35-53.

Index